Living with
dementia

JOHN RIORDAN and BOB WHITMORE

Manchester University Press

Manchester and New York

Distributed exclusively in the USA and Canada
by St. Martin's Press

Published by Manchester University Press
Oxford Road, Manchester M13 9PL, UK
and Room 400, 175 Fifth Avenue,
New York, NY 10010, USA

Distributed exclusively in the USA and Canada
by St. Martin's Press, Inc.,
175 Fifth Avenue, New York, NY 10010, USA

British Library cataloguing in publication data
Riordan, John
    Living with dementia—(Professional self-help guides).
    1. Man. Neuroses: Anxiety
    I. Title II. Whitmore, Bob III. Series
    618.97'68983

Library of Congress cataloging in publication data
Riordan, John.
    Living with dementia.
    (Living with—)
    Includes bibliographical references.
    1. Senile dementia. I. Whitmore, Bob. II. Title
III. Series. [DNLM: 1. Dementia, Senile. 2. Health
Services for the Aged. WT 150 R585L]
RC524.R56   1990 618.97'68983   88-27359

ISBN 0 7190 2515 X *hardback*
ISBN 0 7190 2516 8 *paperback*

Typeset in New Century Schoolbook
by Koinonia, Manchester
Printed in Great Britain
by Bell & Bain Ltd., Glasgow

Contents

Preface

As the title of this book suggests, it has been written for both carers and for professionals who may be involved in services for elderly people. We both work with individual elderly people and their families, and we are also involved in regular staff-training programmes. The basic content of the book is based on our experience in these areas, and we've tried to answer some of the questions that have come up in the course of our work. We are members of families ourselves, and have elderly relatives, some of whom have suffered from dementia; and these experiences have affected the content of the book significantly.

We hope it is not an 'advice' book – we've often found that the last thing carers need is advice. We have found that they are often in great need of information, practical assistance, and a listening ear. We can't provide the last two, so have concentrated on providing relevant information., This information does include a description of the feelings experienced by many carers, and we hope this will be of help to those carers who often feel isolated and alone.

Professionals likewise will find at least some of the chapters helpful in terms of summarising some of the basic knowledge of dementia, as well as giving a flavour of the experience of carers and elderly people. We feel this is important as it is often easy for professionals to get lost in the technical problems of dealing with dementia, and to forget about the feelings of those whose care often adds up to twenty-four hours a day, as well as the feelings of elderly confused people themselves. We have tried to place this information in the context of the society we live in today, for as we will see, society itself is changing in ways which profoundly affect how we see old age and consequently how we respond to the needs of elderly people, including those suffering from dementia.

John Riordan
Bob Whitmore

Acknowledgements

Our thanks go to the following for their comments on an earlier draft of this book: Brenda Bramhall, Tim Backhouse, Evelyn Taylor and Paul Markman. Special acknowledgement goes to the members of the Eccles Carers Group who suggested a number of very useful modifications, and to Anne Riordan for her continual editing. Thanks also go to Pamela Sykes for her limitless patience and secretarial skill, and finally to the many elderly people and their carers in the Bolton and Eccles areas whose experiences make up the core of this book and the initial impetus for writing it.

1 Elderly people and society

Introduction

Today people are living to a greater age and in greater numbers than ever before. Improvements in social conditions, such as better housing, education, sanitation and welfare payments, and better medical treatment of previously fatal diseases, has meant that people are living longer and more healthy lives. This could be said to be one of the great achievements in public welfare in this century.

There are nearly nine million people over the age of sixty-five in the UK and this represents some 16 per cent of the entire population. This compares to 1.8 million or just 5 per cent of the population in 1900. This trend to an increasingly 'elderly' population is true of nearly all the rich industrial nations and is set to continue. The number of elderly people in our society is likely to increase further. In fact, the number of people over the age of seventy-five is rising most rapidly and is likely to reach about four million by 1996: an increase of 30 per cent in two decades.

Contrary to popular belief most of these elderly people are in perfectly reasonable health. Only a tiny minority are in institutions, two out of three have no, or only slight, disability and three out of four suffer no psychiatric or mental disturbance. Most elderly people can expect to age successfully and never come into contact with social or other services either because they have no need or because they can rely on the informal support of family or friends if such a need arises. It is important to understand at the outset that dementia is a problem for only a minority of elderly people. Widespread prejudices linking old age and 'senility' are just not true of the experiences of the majority of people in their later years. As we shall see, the problems posed by dementia for families and society at large are great enough without their being exaggerated.

The problem of dementia

Unfortunately, too often the problems of elderly people are met with a hysterical response by some commentators. There are fears that the burden caused by illnesses like dementia in old age will be too great for society to bear, that the great achievement of longer life is in fact a 'time bomb' of dependency and that elderly people will increasingly 'clog up' our hospitals and social services.

It is certainly true that awareness by both the public and professionals of dementia as a health problem has increased greatly and that the **absolute** number of dementia sufferers, despite the fact that they are a small minority of elderly people, is large and will increase as the population grows older. Some 5 to 8 per cent of those over sixty-five will be seriously affected by dementia and no less than 20 per cent of those over eighty will be similarly affected. So up to one million people in the UK have dementia and require help and care. This is a very large number and indicates the scale of the problems faced not just by the health and social services but by ordinary people and families.

Dementia is now an issue of great concern and interest. In the past all kinds of brain disorders in old people were given the blanket name 'senility'. Nowadays, it is recognised that dementia is not one but a number of different diseases which can be distinguished from one another and, at least in theory, are potentially treatable if the causes of them can be found (see Chapter 4). Recently new health and social services have developed to meet more of the needs of sufferers. The type of help available varies considerably from place to place but includes home visiting services, day centres and hospitals and different kinds of residential care. These services will be discussed in Chapter 8. However, the vast majority of elderly people live in their own homes and are maintained in the community by their family, usually by female relatives on whom the duty of this kind of care conventionally falls. This care, by wives, daughters and daughters-in-law, but also by husbands and more rarely sons, can be lonely, stressful and unremitting. In recent years a new emphasis has been placed on community care by successive governments but it is by no means clear whether the help and support that families need is being more successfully delivered.

Assumptions about old age

To understand the problems of dementia fully, we have to start at the concept of 'old age' itself and examine how the old fit in to our current society and the kind of assumptions that are made about them. The first point to understand is that 'old age' is an idea which arises out of culture not biology. A man does not undergo any noteworthy physical or biological changes, on reaching the age of sixty-five, which mark him out from someone a couple of years younger. What does mark him out is the fact that society has 'retired' him and from that point (sixty-five years of age, or sixty for a woman) he will officially be considered as part of the elderly population, notwithstanding his own views on the matter. He will be in receipt of a pension and, unless he has made private arrangements, will depend on the state for his income and care. It must be noted that these 'retirement' ages are completely arbitrary and were chosen for political and economic reasons when retirement pensions were first introduced in the early part of this century. They could, and probably will, be changed in the future, most likely in a downward direction, reflecting trends to 'early retirement'. There could be a number of reasons for this, the most significant being perhaps the need for governments to increase the number of jobs available by effectively forcing people to retire early. (Retired people of course are not included in unemployment statistics.)

Once retired, elderly people officially become, along with children and the long-term disabled, part of the 'dependent' population; that is, dependent on the state for income and health care. As a group, they tend to be rather poor. Statistically they are likely to be living in the poorest housing, often alone, and frequently on the poverty line. Public awareness of these facts reaches a height during cold spells when the problem of old people dying from cold reveals the penury and misery many are reduced to. It seems a paradox that, at a time when many more people are living longer lives, the quality of those remaining years becomes poorer and old age itself is less valued than in non-industrial societies.

Modern society is characterised by rapid technological development, to the extent that middle-aged and older people may find their skills and experiences completely outdated within their life-span. This is rapidly becoming a feature of industrialised nations. Loss of role, sense of purpose and self-esteem are often consequences of removal from the labour market, along with excessive free time, and the feeling that society no longer wants any contribution from you.

To be old is to carry a certain stigma, as can be seen by looking at things which are highly valued in our society: youth, health, beauty, novelty, sexuality, wealth, productivity, physical fitness, energy, 'go-getting' and independence. These are not values associated with old age. Although there is little basis for these assumptions, the advantages of age, such as wisdom, judgement and long experience from the past, are not as respected as they once were and still are in other countries. It is not surprising, in such a society, that elderly people do not fit in with the mainstream of the culture, but seem rather a burden, faintly ridiculous and out of touch with reality. Some of the most common assumptions about them are that:

1 they are sick and diseased;
2 they are better off with their own kind;
3 they require **rest** and peace;
4 they can't cope with change ('you can't teach an old dog new tricks').

Old age and disease. It cannot be denied that a relationship between old age and disease does exist. As people get older they are more prone to chronic degenerative diseases such as dementia. Other examples of chronic illnesses which are more common in elderly people are arthritis, diabetes, high blood pressure and rheumatism. It is estimated that one in eight of the population aged sixty-five and over has a severe disability and that a further one in four has some moderate disablement. Therefore some three million elderly people will have some measure of disability.

However, for many hundreds of years, old age was itself viewed as a kind of incurable disease for which it was hoped a single cause would one day be found. Various theories as to the causes of old age were put forward at certain times including the view that it was due to degeneration of the arteries (arteriosclerosis) – an idea that still has some currency today, as is illustrated by the common expression 'hardening of the arteries' which is used to explain all manner of debility in the elderly. A number of more exotic theories were also popular from time to time including a theory which held that the decay of the sex glands was central to the ageing process, which led an eminent French doctor to inject himself with a preparation made from animals' testicles in the hope of slowing down his own ageing, needless to say without any noticeable result. Similarly, in the United States today some scientists are using themselves as experimental subjects in the hope that they will be able to demonstrate that the daily intake of certain vitamins postpones the ageing process. Modern science no longer claims that biological ageing has a given cause. Today ageing is regarded as an inherent part of the life process, as an inevitable and natural stage in the development of all living things. However, the long history which has seen old age as a variant of sickness and disease has had a powerful influence on our institutions and policies for the aged and on our assumptions about old people.

The major charities for the elderly, 'Age **Concern**' and '**Help** the Aged', by their very titles express a strong image of old age as a pitiable time. It is thought to be good practice to have nurses employed in private rest homes even though none of the residents may be sick. Many residential homes will be run by ex-nurses. Some will still have 'matrons' in charge, special clinic rooms, drug cupboards and other hospital paraphernalia. Elderly people may be driven to the local day centres in ambulances despite being in perfectly good health. 'Old age' is still used as a diagnosis by some doctors. It is still too common for elderly people to be told 'your problem is old age', or 'what do you expect at your age?', or 'wouldn't you be better off in a home at your age?' The words 'old and frail', 'old and infirm', 'old and senile' trip naturally off the tongue.

In general the connection between old age and disease remains uppermost in the public's mind. Yet, we have already noted that the vast majority of elderly people in this country are not in need of care and are in reasonably good health. Even in those people aged seventy-five and over, whose risk of disablement from chronic diseases like dementia is greatest, almost half report no, or only slight, disablement.

'Elderly people are better off with their own kind'. One of the most common assumptions about elderly people is that they are better off with their own kind. In Britain there is a well-established tradition of segregated facilities for the old: nursing homes, rest homes, old people's homes, sheltered flats, retirement communities. The value of segregation does not seem in question. Throughout life there is undoubtedly a common bond with our particular generation. We have grown up in the same era, been subject to the same influences and developments. However, as adults we have contact with and access to people of all ages and backgrounds. There seems little reason to suppose that elderly people prefer to be with their own. In fact many octogenarians do not consider themselves to be old and neither do they like to mix with 'old people'.

There are cost and convenience advantages to gathering old people together where they can be 'looked after' in a safe environment where resources are 'efficiently' used. The danger of segregation is that it may foster an attitude of 'out of sight, out of mind'. There may be a certain benefit to society in having painful problems like old age, illness or disease removed from its midst and safely disposed. Admissions to institutions for the aged too often means no possibility of further treatment or active therapy even though a proportion of those admitted have conditions which are potentially reversible or treatable.

Many of these segregated services for elderly people were set up with the best of intentions. For example, the aims of the 1948 National Assistance Act, which created local authority old people's homes, were very laudable. Prior to the Act provision for the elderly, including those with dementia, had been linked to the care of the poor and socially rejected. The new homes would do away with the stigma of the workhouse and would be, in the words of the Minister for Health (Nye Bevin), 'hotels for the working classes'. Old people, who had made their contributions to society, would come for a restful and well-serviced old age. But the record of these segregated, and often semi-closed, institutions is not a good one. For example, numerous studies have been carried out on old people's homes since their inception, nearly all of which indicate that admission to such a home is equivalent to social death. More recently there has been widespread concern about standards of care in private nursing homes following media exposés and personal recantations from former staff concerning the abuse and exploitation of residents, including substandard food, misuse of drugs, fire risks, and physical and mental abuse. In turn the local authorities, given the responsibility to register and monitor all private residential homes in the Residential Homes Act (1984), are in a weak position, being unable to insist on standards which their own residential establishments may fail to meet.

The assumption that segregated facilities are best for old people and essential for those with major disabilities is being questioned. Alternative forms of help are necessary which maintain the independence of elderly people and enable them to stay in their familiar environment.

Rest and peace. It is a widespread belief that what elderly people want is rest and peace, away from the striving and competition of the youthful world, where they can enter into contemplation and reminisce on their past lives. According to this view old people are happy with little activity or social contact as they withdraw from an outer to an inner orientation. It is natural for them to meditate on their past lives and to release themselves from responsibilities, commitments and ties of family affections. During the 1960s this idea was given the name of 'disengagement' by some research workers. Disengagement is a kind of psychological preparation for death. Successful ageing is said to depend on the extent to which an elderly person achieves this disengagement in his or her later years.

The effects of this belief can also be seen in places where elderly people are brought together, such as **rest** homes, old people's homes and hospitals. Such places may be 'off the beaten track' or tucked away in quiet cul-de-sacs and often have a monastic feel to them. There may be an emphasis on quiet, on lack of activity and excitement, on minimal contact with the surrounding community and on images of rest and peace, such as flowers (perhaps left over from a previous funeral), cleanliness and immaculate order. The names of such buildings often contain horticultural imagery, for example, *White Meadows, Oaklands, Riverside, Beechfield, Conifers, Greenacres* and so on. They may even be situated in uncannily close proximity to local cemeteries and crematoria. Once entered, few elderly people will leave such places.

The theory of disengagement has some convenient consequences. It means, for example, that there is a minimal need for expensive services, activities and leisure facilities for the aged. Another theory suggests that the lack of stimulation and social contact evident in many institutions is preferred by old people and is therefore nothing to worry about. All elderly people want, according to this theory, is to be left alone.

There is very little evidence that rest and peace is 'natural' in the elderly. Surveys in a number of countries have found that there is very little decline in the range and number of activities of even the oldest people, given a reasonable level of income and good health; nor is there much indication, from the way the clubs, day centres and meeting places are used, that elderly people are withdrawn, want to be alone and are preparing for death. These assumptions carry very negative consequences for older people and are just not supported by any evidence we have available.

They can't cope with change. It is true that elderly people on average have somewhat more difficulty in learning new things than younger people and that, because of other changes in the body that occur as people get older, they cannot react as quickly to events and show a reduced speed of response. However, this does not mean that elderly people cannot learn or adapt to change, or that they are rigid and inflexible.

There has been a great deal of scientific interest in what elderly people can do compared with younger people, both on the part of psychologists and others. For example, after the last war when labour was scarce, research programmes were set up to investigate the capabilities of the older worker. Such studies have usually taken place in research laboratories and it is not clear how results of tests in such artificial surroundings relate to actual performance in real life. In practical studies in real life situations there is little to suggest mental decline. For example, the research into older workers did show that on average it took them a little longer to learn new things but it also showed that elderly workers operated well within their abilities and therefore had no problem at all. This will be a great relief to many doctors, members of parliament, judges, not to mention members of the House of Lords, many of whom are in their seventies, eighties and beyond and performing perfectly well in their work. Winston Churchill was sixty-five years old on becoming Prime Minister in 1939. Mrs Thatcher is sixty-two years old at the time of writing and there is no suggestion that she is unable to cope with change. President François Mitterrand has been re-elected President of France at the age of seventy-one.

Of course these are all rather special people, but the experience of many elderly people is of change and transition. Some of these changes are rather negative ones such as the onset of a disabling illness or the death of a spouse, but if anything, elderly people have been shown to be better at dealing with these kinds of stresses than younger people.

The effects of ageism

These beliefs about old age are examples of 'ageism'. This is a generalised negative attitude towards the elderly, based on untruths or partial truth, which is held by large numbers of the general public. Such an attitude may arise from fear or lack of knowledge. Unjustified beliefs about old age are also held by many elderly people. Often people in their seventies and eighties will vehemently deny being 'old' as if to be so called is a term of abuse. Ageism affects the quality of life of all elderly people. There is a danger of the old entering a spiral of dependency (Figure 1.1) which, at least in part, is created by the way in which society treats older people. Low expectations from others and the lack of a role add to the other real pressures that exist, such as reduced income and poor health. It is likely that the vast majority of the elderly avoid the harshest effects of these attitudes as long as they stay relatively independent and in good health. But those with handicaps and disabilities are brought face to face with them in many of our services for the old.

Ageism and dementia. Although dementia does occur occasionally in younger persons (and this may increase in the future because of the spread of AIDS) it is primarily elderly people who are affected and who live with the consequences of the disease. Dementia occurs (largely) within the context of old age. Hostile attitudes towards old age make it more likely that especially troublesome behaviour shown by an elderly person will be tolerated less well by those around them. Pressure to have elderly people with dementia admitted to long-stay residential care, which may not be in their best interest, is an example of this. There is also a tendency for any difficult behaviour in an elderly person to be 'labelled' negatively. For example, what passes for determination in a young person, is labelled 'cranki-

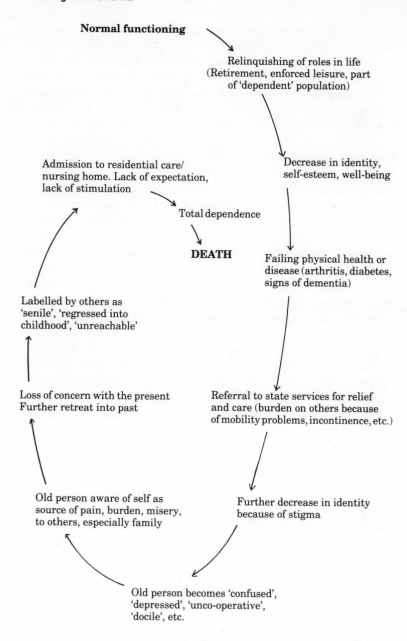

Figure 1.1 The spiral of dependency in old age

ness' in an older person., What, in a 30-year-old, is 'forgetful-ness', becomes evidence of senility in an 80-year-old.

Dementia is a serious disease and a major cause of disability and death in elderly people. There is no cure and little can be done to stop the illness itself. However, much can be done to prevent the additional powerful handicaps which are imposed on sufferers as a result of insufficient support, low expectations, hostile attitudes and fear. Unfortunately all of the assumptions we have considered here are applied with more force to people with dementia which is a disease still regarded by many as just ageing in a rather more extreme form. Thus, those with demen-tia are very likely to be segregated, within homes and places for the old, into special 'wings' and units, minimising their contact with other so-called rational people. They are likely to be viewed as completely 'disengaged', living in their own private world of incoherent thoughts and past events, and incapable of express-ing their needs. They may be seen as completely incapable of adapting to, or even reacting to, change. Finally, they may be considered to be already dead as personalities albeit in a living body.

We make these points to illustrate the variety of factors which operate on elderly people and to draw the reader's attention to the fact that dementia is more than just a biological process. Dementia is a social, as well as medical, problem and cannot really be divorced from attitudes and policies which affect elderly people in general.

The policy of community care

One of the most important policies affecting elderly people and their families is 'community care'. The policy states that, as far as possible, old people should be allowed to remain in their own homes and their needs met within their natural communities rather than in institutions such as long-stay hospitals and local authority homes. These ideas are not new, in fact community care has been the official policy of successive governments since the late 1950s.

Care by the community has always been the only care that most elderly people in need are likely to receive. Ninety-five per cent of all elderly people, and 80 per cent of dementia sufferers, live in private households. The great majority of these people receive no state services and are managing by themselves or with the help of family or friends. A problem arises, however, in that the vast bulk of resources for elderly people is spent on residential and institutional services and there is widespread agreement that state support for those at home is, at best, patchy and inadequate.

It is only during this century that old people have received any special care at all, such as pensions, allowances and state-sponsored services like day centres and residential homes. Prior to this, they depended on various charitable concerns and the workhouse. It is quite true that there was no 'golden age' for elderly people. In the past people were left to fend for themselves in a society where you worked until you dropped. Those elderly people who became ill, frail or senile shared their fate with vagrants, tramps, prostitutes, orphans, the mentally ill and other social casualties. Old people who needed care received either 'outdoor relief' from their local parish or confinement in a workhouse.

The workhouse system continued until the Local Government Act of 1929 and the stigma and shame attached to it still live on in the memories of many elderly people, despite the fact that many modifications were made to it over the years. It developed from a system of deterrent institutions into an instrument of social welfare combining the roles of school, hospital, asylum, old people's home and last refuge. But the services it provided were not very good. The buildings were formidable, impersonal, and prison-like, and institutionalisation was promoted to the extent that routines became an end in themselves and human relationships were distorted and destroyed.

Following the introduction of the National Health Service (1948) and old people's homes (1947) criticism of institutions for the aged continued. This was because many of the buildings and practices of the pre-war institutions were still used in the new system. (The current pattern of residential provision for the elderly is described in Chapter 9). The following issues have provoked particular concern: the extent to which human rights and dignity have or have not been protected in residential care; the segregated nature of such services; the geographical remoteness and lack of access to many of them; the lack of physical and social connection with surrounding communities; the lack of choice experienced by residents/patients; the lack of participation; and the lack of activities, stimulation and human contact. Because of these problems and following failures to correct them in residential services, the trend over the last thirty years has been for institutional care to be seen as a last resort, even for severely disabled people, and governments have placed a new emphasis on community care. In practice this means keeping elderly people in their own homes for longer periods or for as long as possible.

Of course the policy of community care also has its problems. For example, the extent to which the community is either caring, or even interested in the problems caused by dementia, has been doubted by some commentators. Others think that the social conditions which may once have promoted neighbourly and family care are changing fast.

Caring communities? A caring community would be one that showed good neighbourliness, a tolerance for disordered behaviour, an interest in what happens to its individual members, a network of social contact and voluntary 'giving' (in time and energy) to an elderly person suffering from dementia. Yet we know that in the vast majority of cases it is relatives alone who give this support and that the involvement of outside agencies or the 'community' is minimal. Therefore community care is, in fact, care by relatives. It might be morally good for the nation that ordinary people be involved personally on a voluntary basis, in the care of unrelated people who are sick or needy and it is sometimes claimed that such a sense of community existed in the past. But there is not much evidence that such neighbourly support is very widespread today; in fact many of the values in our society may militate against it. Fear of old age, ageism, denial and avoidance of suffering, rampant individualism and a preoccupation with material values and self-fulfilment are all obstacles to the creation of genuinely caring communities. They cannot be legislated for. The end result is that dementia becomes someone else's private grief and responsibility.

Changes in society. Other problems for the policy of community care arise from changes in society which make the delivery of care to elderly people by their relatives more difficult.

For example, there are less children around to care for their elderly parents than there used to be. This is because for a long time people have been having fewer children. Almost a third of all elderly people now live alone. The vast majority of them are women who have outlived their husbands. An increasing number of them have little or no contact with relatives or friends either because they have none or because they are geographically distant from them. Care for older relatives is also affected by divorce and re-marriage which may undermine stable family relationships especially with caring in-law relatives.

The changing position of women in society is also crucial to the policy of community care. The duty of looking after an elderly relative has conventionally fallen on the women in the family, even to the extent that a married woman may well be expected to care for an elderly mother or father-in-law. The bulk of community care is therefore carried out by women. It is estimated that there are over one million people in Britain caring for an elderly person in this way. A typical carer is likely to be a middle-aged married daughter, perhaps with a teenage family and a number of other competing responsibilities. We know that in the UK two thirds of women aged between thirty-five and fifty-four now work at least part-time. Their work is often an essential part of the household earnings. A woman in this position may well be expected to continue working **and** care for an elderly relative **and** bring up a family **and** look after the house. Taking on so many roles can produce intolerable stress and, unless sufficient practical, financial and emotional support is available it is likely to lead to health problems in the carer.

The idea that it is natural for a woman to assume the role of carer for a sick or disabled relative seems generally accepted. A man looking after a disabled person is respected and admired and is likely to receive more of the state supports (like home help) that are available, than a woman carer in a similar position. The fact that women are now eligible for an invalid care allowance, (see Chapter 8) on an equal footing with men, is a major break through, although it must be remembered that the case had to go before the European Court of Human Rights before this victory for women was achieved.

Conclusion

It has been claimed that community care is popular with governments because by promoting it, they make considerable cost savings. However, even from this brief discussion of the policy, one can see that community care for the elderly is never likely to be a cheap option. Dementia sufferers in particular often require intensive support in order to be maintained in the community and the fact that the vast majority **are** maintained in the community is a testimony to the extent of family care they are receiving. Nevertheless, help, advice and relief from the stress of caring are often needed by families supporting an elderly relative with dementia. For most of them help from the state services only marginally touches on these problems. In this sense, the promises of the community care policy have yet to be honoured. However, it is also true that the extent of need generated by a problem like dementia can never be met by the state alone. Voluntary activity by individuals and groups, personal inconvenience and self-sacrifice, courage in the face of great age, mental disorder and suffering, are the types of qualities needed to create a society which is able to cope effectively with dementia.

Summary

1 The number of elderly people in the population has shown a marked increase this century. However this development is often regarded with alarm rather than with a sense of achievement.

2 Unwarranted assumptions and attitudes about old age are commonplace, are reflected in our services for the elderly and are very damaging to the lives of old people.

3 The majority of elderly people age successfully. Only a minority are affected by chronic illness and diseases like dementia.

4 Dementia is a source of great concern because the number of sufferers will increase as the population grows older. Five to 8 per cent of people over the age of sixty-five have dementia and more than 20 per cent of those aged eighty and over are similarly affected.

5 Dementia is not just a biological problem. It is a social problem and cannot be separated from attitudes and policies which affect elderly people in general.

6 'Community care' is the current social policy likely to have most

impact on elderly people and dementia sufferers. It is, to a large extent, a response to long-standing criticisms of institutional care for the aged.

7 The promises of community care have yet to be kept. Practical, emotional and financial support for families and carers is patchy and inadequate. The bulk of resources continue to be directed towards residential care for the elderly – both public and (especially under the current government) private.

8 Taking care of seriously disabled elderly people in their own homes is never likely to be a cheap or easy option.

2 The experience of dementia

This chapter is an attempt to describe the feelings of an elderly person who is suffering from confusion due to dementia. It is based on our experience of working with people who are confused, and we have tried to 'get in the shoes' of an elderly woman in order to describe some aspects of her life. Although it is just an imaginary case, we hope that it captures a little of the sense of what it might be like to be confused.

Amy is seventy-eight years old and has recently moved in with her daughter, Jenny, her husband, John, and family (17-year-old David and 19-year-old Debbie). She lived by herself previously, her husband Jim having died nine years ago. She moved to her daughter's because she was becoming increasingly forgetful and isolated.

'I wake up, and my first feeling is worry. I have a feeling that I should be up and doing something. I can't quite get hold of what it should be. It's like that feeling when you know you've made a mental note to do something, but can't for the life of you remember what. It's like that but much worse. I get up and it's still dark – but then I've been used to getting up when it's dark all my life – and I go downstairs. I'm not sure whether to dress or not. I find myself in the kitchen, and I'm reminded that I should be making breakfast. I open the cupboards and look for pots and pans, but the kitchen is not like mine, and for a few moments I feel panicky as I don't know whose house I'm in. Have I just wandered into someone else's? What will they do when they find me? I hear a voice shouting "Mum!" The voice is tired and cross. I suddenly remember it's my daughter, Jenny, and I'm staying with her. I can't remember why or for how long. She comes into the kitchen in her dressing gown. "Mum, what are you doing down here again? Don't you know what time it is? It's nearly four in the morning! Come on, I'll take you upstairs." I feel so foolish, and embarrassed – I'd just forgotten. I can remember Jenny as a child so well, and now here she is looking at me as though I'm a fool, and she herself looks worn and tired. She takes me back to the bedroom (it doesn't seem much like **my** bedroom) and I go to bed, and try to remember the old days, when I used to be up at six to get my husband off to work, before I started to get everything ready for the day. For a few seconds I can't remember his name – and I feel that panic rising – not even remembering my own husband's name! I can picture him so easily, but his name has disappeared into a jumble of words. Jim! It eventually pops up into my head, and I feel relieved – I'm not going completely gaga yet!

'Jenny wakes me up in the morning, and tells me, "I couldn't get back to sleep after last night". I don't know what she's talking about, and so I just look at her. I've a feeling that I've done something wrong, and I feel cross that she should make me feel this way. I haven't even got up yet. "Don't you remember what you did last night?!" I say "Oh Jenny, behave yourself!" This makes me feel better for a second. I can talk to her like she is a child as well. But she gets angry and tells me how I got up in the middle of the night and clattered around the kitchen waking everyone up. I can't remember, and it feels bad to be blamed for something you can't even remember doing. And it feels bad not to remember. My memory is shocking. I can remember things that happened twenty, thirty or fifty years ago as if they were yesterday, but I forget everything that did happen yesterday – or even today. I feel this panic in the background all the time. Can you imagine what it's like to forget what you are doing all the time. I feel like I am walking on a tightrope all day. If I slip I will fall into this jumble of confusion, where nothing makes any sense, and never will again.

'Sometimes I feel fine though. Last week (I think!) Jenny and I made some bread together. I used to make the family bread of course, and I taught Jenny how to, though she never made bread after she got married. She got all the ingredients out for me (I'd never find them in this kitchen of hers!) and once I got started, my hands seemed to know what to do. I did forget whether I'd put the salt in though, and Jenny had to stop me putting two lots in. We had a laugh about that, though at first I felt that panicky feeling rising. It was nice when we had it for tea, and the family told me how delicious it was. I'd like to do more cooking, but Jenny gets cross with me sometimes, as I like to do things my way, and I feel silly if I get stuck, and don't want to ask her for help. Sometimes, like with the bread, its alright though. At times I feel nervous when we have dinner together. Jenny's children talk so fast I can't seem to follow what they're saying. I'm a bit deaf as well so I have to concentrate to hear them. Today I shouted at David who's the youngest (I forget how old he is, but he's a strapping teenager now). I can't remember what he was saying, but he was going on at his sister Debbie about some record or other, and it just got too much for me so I told him to shut up. Everybody went quiet, and though I felt better, I suddenly felt nervous. I'll get put away if I do things like that. It was alright though and everybody laughed after. Except David who glared at me for the rest of the meal, but I'm used to that with naughty children.

'Debbie's a love though. We had a nice chat a while ago about what things were like before her mother was born. She's at college now. I can't remember what she is studying but she wanted to know about life after the war. Jenny got my photo album out, and looking at the pictures reminded me of so much. I could have talked for hours. It was lovely to remember those times, even though some were very hard, and seeing photographs of Jenny and Brian when they were little, and then as they got older made me feel, well, secure. They are part of me, and their children too. It's that feeling secure that I don't have as much these days. It's difficult being secure on a tightrope. And I wonder where the tightrope is going sometimes.

'I can't remember when, but I know it wasn't too long ago that I woke up in the morning and found that I'd wet the bed. I just wanted to die. A grown woman wetting her bed like a baby. If I could, I would just have given up and died right there. Jenny didn't say anything but I could tell from her face what she was thinking, as she took the sheets downstairs to be washed. I cried, but Jenny talked to me about it later on. I felt so guilty and embarrassed though. Wetting my own bed at my age. I can't remember much what Jenny said, but I don't have so much to drink at night now. She's also got some pads which I suppose are for the bed, though I don't want them. I've not done it again so I hope I won't have to have them. I don't want to go into a home. I don't want to sit all day with a lot of old people doing nothing. I can help Jenny here. Although she gets upset with me at times (sometimes I think my awful memory upsets her more than it does me!) we do get on well overall. It is a tightrope though. Sometimes, like when I helped make the bread, and when I talked to Debbie, the tightrope is nice and thick, and I feel secure.

At other times it's so thin, and I feel so panicky. I know that thinking about the past can help me to feel more secure, but I don't want to live in the past. I know I can't remember as much, and I do silly things at times, but I can still do some things, even if I need help. And I have all these memories – I can see these changes, and the things which don't change. I can talk about this – if people ask me.'

This account illustrates a few important points about confusion which are worth examining in more detail.

Firstly, the confused person is **aware** that he or she is confused. The feelings of fear this creates must be very powerful. We've probably all experienced very brief episodes of confusion: those first few seconds on waking up in a strange place; or after fainting; or even when we've had too much to drink. For a person who is experiencing confusion this feeling will be present all the time, although it will vary in intensity. Similarly, we all forget things, but to forget things continually must be very distressing. These feelings of fear and distress are of course very understandable, but it does seem that people who live and/or work with elderly people who are confused often do not appreciate the strength of these feelings.

Secondly, if we look at the account of Amy, she describes these feelings as 'walking on a tightrope'. To put it another way, her sense of **control** is very vulnerable. We all feel a bit vulnerable if we find ourselves, for example, in a strange place or in situations where we do not know anybody. It's as if knowing a place gives us a sense of control which helps our sense of security. In situations where we feel vulnerable we have to rely on our own resources, such as our sense of purpose. If we are confused those resources are reduced. Confused people therefore have less control over the **external** world, but, and far worse than this, their sense of control over their **internal** world – their own mind – is shaken as well, as they cannot rely on memory.

This loss of control can best be described as a sense of **helplessness** which occurs if we have little or no power to affect things. The sense of helplessness is particularly significant with elderly confused people who have lost a lot of control in their lives. If helplessness becomes overwhelming, people can just give up. In Amy's case her incontinence (loss of control over her own body) led to powerful feelings of helplessness such that she wanted to give up and die at the time.

Looking back at Amy's story we can see that the experiences which are most positive involve her sense of **control** being supported. Making bread and looking at her photos with Debbie are both experiences which increase her control, and therefore her security.

Finally, confused people may also **deny** being forgetful. Because it can be so **painful** to admit (to yourself and other people) that you are confused, a better way of dealing with it seems to be to deny it altogether. Although Amy does not deal with her confusion in this way, it is quite common, and is in some ways an understandable way of dealing with distress. (We will look at this in more detail in Chapter 6.)

Summary

1 Confusion and memory loss are bound to lead to very powerful and negative feelings on the part of sufferers, although people who live and/or work with elderly, confused people may not recognise the extent of this.
2 People who are suffering memory loss will be only too aware of this although they may deny it or find it very hard to discuss. They will also experience very powerful feelings of fear about what is happening, and about what **will** happen to them.
3 Confusion and memory loss are likely to lead to loss of control and feelings of helplessness. So the things that elderly people **can** still do are extremely important in order to compensate for the things they **cannot** do anymore.

3 The clinical picture of dementia

Introduction

In the last chapter we tried to put ourselves 'in the shoes' of an elderly person with dementia and imagined how painful and difficult the realisation must be that something is wrong with one's ability to think. Now we will examine how dementia appears from an outsider's point of view. What are the problems of behaviour and thought which indicate that an old person may be suffering from dementia? These questions are asked both by doctors as they try to make a diagnosis and by relatives as they attempt to make sense of what may be happening to their loved one.

When we say someone is confused we are drawing attention to the fact that a person is unable to think with his or her usual clarity and purpose. All of us will have had some experience of feeling 'confused' and what we usually mean by this is some brief moment of bewilderment or lack of clarity: an inability to solve a puzzle or understand instructions or follow a plot. The confusion we experience on these occasions demands an explanation. It is a sign of something else which is affecting us: distraction, anxiety, anger or just plain stupidity. Similarly, we take confusion in an elderly person as a sign of some deep-rooted problem such as an illness or a disease which is affecting their ability to think and make sense of their surroundings. But **here** we are not talking of some brief moment but of a confusion which is indefinitely prolonged, which involves not just thought but also the emotions and behaviour and which arises not just in connection with a complex problem but in response to all manner of simple, routine tasks which should be second nature and which have been performed without difficulty since childhood.

In this more specialised use of the term a person can show confusion in one of two ways. The first of these is called an 'acute confusional state' or **delirium**. The second is known as a 'chronic confusional state' or **dementia**. We will describe each of these in turn.

Acute confusional state (delirium)

An acute confusional state (also called delirium) comes on rapidly within hours or days. It is quite often seen in young children, for example, who develop a fever or high temperature. Elderly people are also rather susceptible to becoming delirious when they are ill. A delirious person typically will show marked changes in their mood and emotions. They may show fearfulness, alarm and anger, and these emotions will fluctuate rapidly. Their speech may become slurred. The content of their speech may be difficult to understand or become nonsensical. Sometimes a delirious person will appear to be hallucinating (seeing or hearing things which are not there) and they will be restless, agitated and unable to recognise their surroundings.

These symptoms will have occurred suddenly, if not 'out of the blue', then over a period of days. The confusion arises usually because of an illness to the body which may or may not be obvious. There are many illnesses which lead to such a reaction especially in old people. Infections are the most common cause. For example, an elderly person with a chest infection, or an infection in the urinary tract, can become confused in this way. Other causes which must be investigated include malnourishment, chronic constipation, alcohol abuse and the side-effects of prescribed drugs (see Chapter 5). Any elderly person showing a confusion of rapid onset should be seen at once by a doctor. Delirium is usually easily treated when the underlying illness causing it is diagnosed.

Chronic confusional state (dementia)

A chronic confusional state, or dementia, is a gradual and general decline in a person's thought and personality over an extended period of time (usually years). An affected person will show an increasing difficulty in remembering, concentrating, learning and speaking coherently. As time goes on their capacity to think declines to the extent that they do not know where they are, who they are with or what they should be doing. They may become incapable of planning an action or carrying out an intention. They may have increasing problems controlling the functions of the body (such as urination) and movement (such as

dressing and walking). Changes in personality occur. For example, a previously lively person may become sullen, moody and
irritable to the point of aggression. Social graces may be lost
leading to rudeness and offensiveness to others, perhaps even to
an inability to distinguish between behaviours which should be
private (like undressing) and those which are socially acceptable
in public. As the disease progresses the personal resources of an
affected individual may be seen to diminish. Inactivity, dullness
and lack of initiative may follow. The rate at which such symptoms develop and their severity will vary from person to person
depending on the nature of the disease causing the dementia, the
personal resources of the sufferer and the amount of support and
care they have available. However, dementia is progressive, that
is, it continues to get worse, leading in time to a total dependence
on others and ultimately to death.

From this account we can see that the changes that take place
in dementia are slow and gradual. Whereas in delirium changes
take place over hours and days, the time course in dementia is
months and years. The onset of dementia may be so gradual that
at first it may be difficult to separate the symptoms from general
changes in the personality of the sufferer. Symptoms of early
dementia may be interpreted by the family as 'crankiness',
'awkwardness', or simply 'old age'. Silly mistakes, such as
putting on odd clothes, making tea in the kettle or mixing up hot
and cold water taps, may cause some alarm, but at first are
isolated and exceptional. In most other respects an elderly
person may seem to be functioning relatively well. However,
such an elderly person may well lose their bearings, apparently
suddenly, when their habits and routines are disrupted by a
change in circumstances, such as a brief period in hospital,
moving house or the death of a supporter. It is important to
remember that, in such cases, these events have not **caused** the
dementia but made it **obvious** by removing the sufferer's habitual ways of coping. These points are illustrated in the following case history.

Mrs Butler was a 79-year-old former school mistress living by
herself in the terraced house where she had brought up her three
sons and where she had lived with her husband until his death
three years previously. Over a period of three years she had
begun to behave in a way which increasingly suggested dementia. Her household became untidy and disordered. She began to

lose or misplace her benefit books and cash quite regularly. She was given to walking around her neighbourhood carrying large amounts of cash on her person. She would switch on her gas cooker and fail to light it and, as often as not, her front door would be open whether she was in or out. Her memory for events that had just happened became very poor. She looked shabby. She would forget what she had done and what she was about to do. This problem was worsened by almost complete deafness, for which hearing aids brought little improvement and which, anyway, she was very reluctant to wear. Communicating with her was therefore very difficult. Finally she was prone to aggressive outbursts and was very reluctant to let outsiders (such as social workers) into her home.

These symptoms appeared gradually, stage by stage, over a long period of time and worsened at first almost imperceptibly and then by leaps and bounds. Mrs Butler had three sons, one of whom lived abroad, the second in a distant part of the country and a third, who unfortunately had lost contact with his mother, who lived locally. From time to time her second son would visit and offer a room in his home for her. Although she would occasionally stay for a short break, Mrs Butler would soon become anxious to return to her own home and would eventually come back. She was unable to shop, did not cook and would not accept any help from the social services. Her survival in the community depended on a number of neighbours and families living close by whom she had known, although often not very well, before her illness. There were three to four such houses where she would call in turn every day and receive food and drink, some attention and shelter. Some neighbours would receive such calls twice – or sometimes more – a day. It was very rare to find Mrs Butler in her own house. Needless to say, her neighbours found her calls an increasing imposition, especially as she appeared 'confused' and was occasionally rude. They felt they were doing someone else's job and that 'something should be done'.

Although she was confused, Mrs Butler was very territorial about her house. Home helps from the local social services offices would call every day but rarely got inside. Attempts at short-term care in a local old people's home ended in failure as she would become very aggressive and abusive if confined. It seemed that, despite all her very considerable problems, Mrs Butler was determined to survive and had created for herself a system of support through her neighbours which, although tenuous, resulted in her receiving enough food, shelter and contact for her to remain independent of statutory services. She seemed to value very highly her freedom and was physically fit. It is to their great credit that these families had been supporting this very awkward and disorientated lady for so long but, by the time they had contacted statutory services, they were nearing the end of their tether.

To relieve the neighbours it was decided to try and introduce a home help into Mrs Butler's home to cook for her five days a week. Feeding Mrs Butler – sometimes several times a day by the most frequently visited neighbours – was the most demanding aspect of her visits. Neighbours now declined to provide food for Mrs Butler in the hope that this would encourage her to accept the services of the home help and meals on wheels. It was felt that this was preferable to neighbours closing their doors on her.

Almost as soon as the plan was put into action, Mrs Butler's world began to fall apart. On one of her walking trips, she had a fall. She was not seriously injured and no bones were broken, but an ambulance was called and she was brought to the casualty department of the local infirmary. Here, bewildered and confused, Mrs Butler reverted to a former pattern of behaviour and became extremely aggressive. Nurses and doctors who were unfamiliar with her and her illness administered major tranquillising medication (see Chapter 5) and she was transferred to a psychiatric hospital. Here she continued on major tranquillisers in order to keep her 'stable' and manageable. The drugs had the desired effect but affected her movement and her ability to walk. They also lowered her level of consciousness with the result that she became inactive and inert.

Because of her aggressive behaviour on the ward, Mrs Butler was kept on major tranquillisers. It was decided that she should return home, but with regular injections of the drug (see Chapter 5). Mrs Butler was discharged after having been in hospital three weeks. On her first night home the police found her wandering the streets in the early hours, dressed only in a nightgown. She was again taken to the casualty department of the local infirmary and from there in due course to the psychiatric hospital. After this second admission to hospital, Mrs Butler's condition deteriorated seriously. She became dull, apathetic and incontinent. She lost her former exuberance and aggressiveness. Within weeks a decision was made that she was incapable of being supported in the community and she was transferred to a long-stay ward on a permanent basis.

We can see in Mrs Butler's story a number of characteristics which are typical of dementia.

Onset. The development of her symptoms is slow and gradual, quite unlike the presentation seen in someone with delirium, where the onset of symptoms is relatively sudden and dramatic. Sometimes it will often seem to relatives that the dementia started abruptly, following the death of a spouse as in Mrs Butler's case, or after an illness or other trauma. Yet closer examination reveals a slow decline which is shown up by such events. For example, the death of Mrs Butler's husband probably made more obvious a dementia which had existed for some time but which escaped notice, because of his care for her.

Memory impairment. This is frequently the earliest sign of dementia, although it must be emphasised that, as we get older, our memories may not be quite as good as they were and that memory lapses alone do not constitute dementia. Mrs Butler's problems start with relatively minor forgetfulness and absent-mindedness (misplacing benefit books and cash, not being able to find things) and progress to more severe and embarrassing memory lapses (leaving the gas on unlit, forgetting what she had done and what she was about to do). Typically, in dementia memory for recent and remote events are both affected, but with memories of past events being preserved for a longer time into the disease. Memory for names is often particularly affected.

Compensation. In the early days of dementia, a sufferer may well try to cover up or compensate for their increasing difficulty in learning anything new. Mrs Butler, for example, does not wear her hearing aid. She may have simply forgotten to wear it. On the other hand deafness may be helpful in presenting a better front to the world and denying the effects of mental decline. Other sufferers may try to plug the gaps in their memories by making things up or giving unconvincing excuses. Another compensation, which is well illustrated in Mrs Butler's case, is to develop a rigid and well-worn routine. Her round of calls to neighbours is an elaborate example of this. However this kind of routine is vulnerable to the slightest change. Mrs Butler's world falls apart with the attempted introduction of home help services. She could not venture outside her routine without losing her bearings completely. As the dementia progresses and mental abilities decline such compensations become more and more ineffective.

Personality change. Alteration in personality is another aspect of dementia and can be particularly distressing for families. Bizarre and uncharacteristic behaviour, such as stealing or shop-lifting, can occur. A tendency to be much less reserved sexually can surprise and shock relatives. Mrs Butler had been a much-respected schoolmistress and was used to being in authority over others. Such characteristics served her well in establishing her contacts with neighbours but we also see in her an exaggeration of these traits into rudeness and aggression.

Further comments on Mrs Butler. Mrs Butler's case teaches us that attempts to help a demented person can lead to a worsening of their condition. It wasn't Mrs Butler who asked for 'action to be taken', it was her neighbours. Mrs Butler's routine worked well for her but in the end it imposed a burden on her neighbours which they were unwilling to tolerate. They felt that she had become 'their responsibility' and that this was unfair when a family existed and there were authorities paid to look after such people.

Within the space of a few weeks those who sought to help Mrs Butler first disrupted her well-established routine and then further aggravated her mental condition by administering powerful sedative drugs. She was discharged on these drugs despite the fact that it was only in hospital that she showed the violent aggression for which she was given them.

As well as illustrating the many problems caused by dementia, Mrs Butler's is a cautionary tale. It shows that where people with dementia are concerned, our interventions need to be very sensitive and individualised.

Reversible or irreversible. To what extent are problems like Mrs Butler's reversible or treatable by medical means? To

Affecting brain indirectly	Infections (e.g. of chest or urine) Chronic constipation Hyperthyroidism Alcohol intoxication Drug side-effects Kidney or liver failure Vitamin deficiency (malnourishment)

Affecting brain directly	Infections of the brain
	   (e.g. meningitis, encephalitis)
	 Injury to the brain
	   (e.g. falls, trauma)
	 Vascular disease (strokes)
	 Tumours and abscesses

Figure 3.1 Some causes of acute confusional states (delirium)

understand this better we must call to mind our initial distinction between acute and chronic confusional states. It is usual for acute confusional states (delirium) to be temporary. The word 'acute' refers to symptoms of a very intense character which either resolve or lead to longer-term problems within a short period of time. The symptoms of delirium are caused by many varied medical conditions some examples of which can be seen in Figure 3.1.

In most cases confusion arising suddenly in connection with such illnesses will respond to treatment or resolve through the spontaneous recovery of the body. However, there are times when illnesses do result in irreversible damage to the brain. This is more likely, for example, if the illness is centred in the brain itself (like a brain tumour or stroke) rather than affecting the brain indirectly, as in the case of chronic constipation or an over-active thyroid (hyperthyroidism). The extent of recovery after a stroke, head injury or brain tumour will depend on the extent and site of damage to the brain. Other conditions, such as chronic malnourishment, alcoholism, and liver failure, can and do lead to irreversible problems if they go untreated for a critical period of time. However, in nearly all cases of delirium and acute confusion, treatment is possible and available with a high likelihood of total or partial recovery.

The situation is reversed when considering chronic confusional states, or dementia. Here in the vast majority of cases the

Reversible	Tumours of the brain Depression Normal-pressure hydrocephalus
Irreversible	Alzheimer's disease Multi-infarct dementia Pick's disease Jakob-Creutzfeldt disease Huntington's chorea

Fig. 3.2 Some causes of chronic confusional states (dementia)

causal conditions are irreversible and no treatment is available. Some of the causes of dementia are described in Figure 3.2.

In a small number of cases a chronic confusional state is reversible or at least its progress can be arrested by medical treatment. Tumours of the brain, for example, can be removed. A type of depression which sometimes presents a clinical picture of dementia may be reversed by psychiatric treatment. Surgical procedures are available for correcting the build up of fluid in the brain known as normal-pressure hydrocephalus. However, dementia arising from such causes is rare. Unfortunately, in the great majority of people who develop dementia, the underlying illness is not reversible by medical treatment. The most likely causes are Alzheimer's disease and Multi-infarct dementia (M.I.D.), about which more will be said in Chapter 4. Together, these two illnesses, either singly or sometimes affecting the same person simultaneously, account for over 90 per cent of all the dementia seen in people over the age of sixty-five years.

The Diagnosis of Dementia

The main function of the doctor, and especially the neurologist, is to separate cases of dementia which are treatable from those which are not. To summarise, we have seen that medical and surgical treatments do exist for causes such as tumours, vitamin deficiencies (especially alcohol vitamin deficiency and malnutrition) and normal-pressure hydrocephalus, and that the psychiatrist also has a part to play in distinguishing which dementias are caused by a type of depression which can also be treated.

Over-medication can also cause a condition which can be mistaken for dementia, especially in an elderly person. More will be said about this in Chapter 5. We have also seen, however, that for the greatest number of dementias, that is, those caused by Alzheimer's disease, Multi-infarct dementia and, much less commonly, Pick's disease, Jakob-Creutzfeldt disease and Huntington's chorea, there are no effective medical treatments.

The truth is that the clinical picture of dementia has many potential medical causes and early detection is crucial in cases where treatment is available. If treatment is not forthcoming then reversible conditions may well become irreversible. Much depends on the individual skill of the physician, neurologist, psychiatrist or neuropsychologist making the diagnosis. The most important technological aid to diagnosis is computerised-axial-tomography (CAT) which allows the brain to be scanned by thousands of X-ray pictures of the head, taking only a few minutes. They are then analysed by computer to give a picture of what is happening in the brain. However, the usefulness of the CAT-scan is limited because, despite being augmented by image-enhancing techniques, it is still not sensitive enough to diagnose the early stages of dementia. The diagnosis of the more serious and more numerous causes of dementia remains a 'diagnosis of exclusion', that is, all other possible causes must be considered first and then systematically excluded. Diagnosis is lengthy, as a valid diagnosis can only be made by demonstrating a deterioration of mental functioning over a period of time. Only at autopsy can medical diagnosis made during the person's life be verified. This is of great importance because the diagnosis of an irreversible dementia can lead to an absence of much active therapy and, in the absence of self-sacrificing relatives, to a high likelihood of institutional care.

Summary

1 Confusion is not a diagnosis but a set of symptoms and signs that someone is not able to think with his or her usual clarity and purpose.
2 Delirium is an intense and dramatic confusional state which comes on rapidly, usually because of a physical illness which may or may not be obvious.

3 Delirium is a very common set of symptoms, especially in elderly people, and can arise from a very large number of possible causes, some serious enough to result in lasting damage; most are easily treatable and leave no lasting effects.

4 Dementia is a gradual and general decline in all thought processes, also affecting the emotions, personality and movements of the body.

5 Dementia is marked by a slow onset, a long time course (five to twelve years), memory impairment, personality change and finally by lethargy, dullness and inactivity. In the latter stages of the disease total dependence on others is likely.

6 The diagnosis of dementia is a diagnosis of exclusion. All the reversible causes must be systematically excluded. It is also lengthy, as it is only valid if deterioration in mental function can be shown over a considerable period of time.

7 Both dementia and delirium can occur in the same person. For example, a dementia sufferer is more likely to show the presence of illness or drug side effects by a sudden worsening in his or her mental condition.

8 Any elderly person showing a confusion of rapid onset, or a sudden deterioration in their mental state, should be seen at once by a doctor.

4 The brain and dementia

Dementia can be a very confusing condition for everyone involved. We have found that many carers feel very much in the dark in terms of knowing what is causing such distressing symptoms as, for example, severe memory loss, personality changes, and incontinence, with medical jargon sometimes only adding to the confusion. We have therefore written this chapter for those who would like to know about the kinds of damage sustained by the brain in dementia, and why this damage causes the symptoms we see in the condition. The brain is of course an enormously complex organ, to the extent that scientists are still a long way from a thorough understanding of it, and so our description will necessarily be greatly simplified. However this description will still be quite technical, and so readers who are less interested in this area may prefer to skip this chapter and go on to the next one.

1. The neuron and neurotransmitters

The neuron. The neuron – also known as the nerve cell – is the basic building block of the human brain. Our bodies contain many neurons of which there are two basic types: afferent neurons which carry information from the outside world via our senses to the brain, and efferent neurons, by which the brain sends messages to the body. But the bulk of neurons are contained in the brain, where it is estimated that they number about one hundred billion.

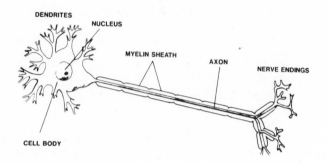

Figure 4.1 The neuron

How the neuron works. The neuron basically works by transmitting information in the form of an electrical impulse. The impulse starts from the nerve endings, passes up through the axon, into the cell body, and then to the dendrites. Figure 4.1 above shows the main features of a typical neuron, although neurons do vary enormously in terms of their size and shape. Some features of the neuron we have not yet mentioned are the myelin sheath, a kind of insulation that surrounds the axon, and the nucleus, which contains the genetic material of the cell.

The dendrites are in contact with the nerve endings of other neurons, although as we shall see later, they do not actually touch. The impulse is triggered in the neuron because of the influence of other neurons whose dendrites are in contact with its nerve endings. If this neuron receives enough impulses from other neurons, the impulse will be triggered and may then cause other neurons it is in contact with to be likewise triggered. The triggering of an impulse is on an 'all or nothing' basis; that is the neuron either receives sufficient stimulation for an impulse to be triggered, or it doesn't – there can be no weak or strong impulses.

As we have suggested, the dendrites of a neuron may be in contact with the nerve endings of many other neurons, and the dendrites of many neurons may be in contact with their own nerve endings. The extraordinary range of mental abilities we all have – our memories, dreams, ideas, consciousness, and so on

– are all due to the relatively simple on-off activity of the many neurons that comprise the brain. However, when we recall that there are about one hundred billion neurons in the brain, the extent of its complexity becomes apparent.

We will shortly describe the sort of damage that is sustained by neurons in dementia, but before this we will look at a crucial aspect involved in the way impulses are transmitted from neuron to neuron – the neurotransmitter. We mentioned previously that the nerve endings and dendrites of the neurons do not actually touch. How then are impulses transmitted from neuron to neuron? The answer is that when an impulse reaches the end of the dendrites, **chemical messengers** are released from the ends, which then pass across the tiny gap between the dendrites of one neuron and the nerve endings of the next. This gap is known as the **synapse**. The chemical messengers land on the nerve endings of the next cell, where they are absorbed into that cell. If enough chemical messengers cross from one (or more) neurons to the next, then the impulse is triggered in that neuron. These vital chemical messengers are known as **neurotransmitters**. In the brain there are a number of different neurotransmitters which tend to be located in specific areas of the brain, and which are involved in different functions. Because neurotransmitters are so crucial for the functioning of the brain, they have been the subject of much research, particularly aimed at relieving disorders which are due to changes in neurotransmitter activity. We will look at this in relation to dementia in the following section.

Neurons, neurotransmitters and dementia. We will now look at the sorts of damage found in neurons in dementia. About one half of elderly persons with dementia have a specific form of the illness known as Senile dementia: Alzheimer's type, sometimes abbreviated to S.D.A.T., and also known more popularly as Alzheimer's disease (Alzheimer is the name of the doctor who first described the illness). When the brains of patients with Alzheimer's disease are studied at post-mortem, two sorts of changes are found in neurons in various places in the brain, Some neurons show tangles of fine fibres **inside** their cell bodies (see Figure 4.1). These are known as **neurofibrillary tangles**, and neurons affected in this way cannot function properly. This is because the tangle prevents, or interferes with, impulses being transmitted. When neurons become further damaged this leads to areas known as **senile plaques**, which are patches of very badly damaged neurons. These areas of damage can occur throughout the brain, but it is in a part of the brain named the **hippocampus** that the damage is most likely to be found. In a following section on the organisation of the brain we will look at the hippocampus in more detail, but we can note at this time that since the hippocampus is involved in memory, damage to its neurons can lead to the severe memory problems found in Alzheimer's disease. The reason why this damage to neurons takes place is still unknown. However, the changes mentioned above also occur in the brains of non-demented elderly people, and this has led to the suggestion that Alzheimer's disease represents an **acceleration** of the normal ageing process. However, there is disagreement amongst scientists about this at the present time.

Since the cause (or causes) of the neurofibrillary tangles and senile plaques are not yet known, we are still some way off finding an effective treatment. One avenue that is being explored involves the neurotransmitters, since again at postmortem the brains of patients with Alzheimer's disease have been found to have abnormalities in certain key neurotransmitters. Although this has led to some hope in terms of a neurotransmitter-based medication, so far no such treatment has been proven to be generally effective.

The changes described above occur in a relatively slow, progressive way, so that the behaviour and functioning of a person with Alzheimer's disease will gradually deteriorate as the neurons in his or her brain are damaged due to an as yet unknown process. However, another major cause of dementia in elderly people lies in disruptions to the blood supply of the brain, so we will look in more detail at this in the following section.

The blood supply to the brain

As we mentioned above, about 50 per cent of elderly people with dementia have the type known as Alzheimer's disease. Another 40 per cent of elderly people with dementia have what is known as multi-infarct dementia, which we will abbreviate to MID. The word 'infarct' simply means an area of dead nerve cells, and so the phrase 'multi-infarct dementia' means dementia brought about by a number of areas of dead cells within the brain. The death of neurons is caused by a loss or reduction of the blood supply to these areas. At this point we should note that the brain gets a very large share of the blood supply. The reason for this lies in the huge number of neurons packed into the brain, and it is such a powerful organ that it is therefore reliant on a rich supply of blood to give it the oxygen and nutrients vital for effective functioning. As a consequence of the need for such a rich blood supply, there is a highly complex and delicate network of arteries and blood vessels which travel to all areas of the brain. We will now look in more detail at multi-infarct dementia.

Multi-infarct dementia. The basic cause of MID is the malfunctioning of blood vessels, for example when they become clogged up with obstructions, such as a piece of debris from a vessel. The effect on the part of the brain that the blood supplies is that the neurons involved die through lack of the oxygen in the blood. It is known that sometimes a blockage is quickly unblocked naturally, in which case the neurons may be temporarily affected through oxygen starvation, but not killed. These temporary blockages are known as transient ischaemic attacks, or TIAs, and the symptoms they produce are temporary. However, in the case of MID, the blockage continues for so long that the neurons die. The reader may at this point note the similarity to the person who has a stroke. In fact many doctors feel that the two conditions are very similar, the difference being when a person suffers a stroke, it is usually a significantly larger area of the brain that is affected, whereas in MID what we see is a **series** of small strokes which gradually disable the patient as their effects multiply. At post-mortem the infarcts appear as tiny holes, the size of a pinhead within the brain.

Multi-infarct dementia and physical illnesses. MID is often related to diseases of the blood supply, such as hypertension (high blood pressure), or problems due to heart conditions. It is also related to 'risk factors' such as smoking, obesity and diabetes.

Neurons in the brain, once destroyed, can never regrow, so the areas of dead cells in MID cannot be treated. However, because of the link with the treatable conditions described above, medication is possible which can reduce the risk of further infarcts, unlike the case of Alzheimer's disease where the cause is still

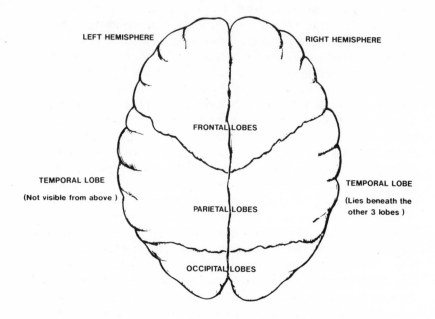

**Figure 4.2 The human brain seen from above showing
the two hemispheres and the lobes**

unknown.

The type of treatment depends upon the nature of the under-lying conditions, so, for example, a patient may be given medication to reduce blood pressure, or to 'thin' the blood, or a heart condition may be treated surgically. Unfortunately treatment may not be feasible, or may be relatively unsuccessful, and so the course of MID in a patient can continue, with the patient deteriorating following each infarct.

We will look at how multi-infarct dementia and Alzheimer's disease differ in a later section in this chapter. In the next section we will go on to look at how the **location** of damage is significant in terms of the **effects** on the person concerned, whether of the type in Alzheimer's disease or multi-infarct dementia.

The organisation of the brain

We have already seen how the brain is packed with neurons. However the brain is of course not just a mass of nerve cells, rather it is organised into a very complex structure, with different areas specialising in doing different things.

In Figure 4.2 above we have a view of the brain as if we are looking down on it from above.

The hemispheres. The first thing to notice is that the brain is split into two halves known as hemispheres. The two hemispheres are in fact joined together by a thick bundle of nerve fibres known as the **corpus callosum**, which is not visible in the diagram. (There are also areas deep in the brain which are not divided into two, and we will be looking at those later.) The two hemispheres tend to specialise in different things: the right hemisphere appears to deal with visual and spatial processing, as well as feelings, intuition and imagination; the left hemisphere deals more with language, logical thinking and calculation. Another feature of the hemispheres is that each is responsible for controlling and receiving information from its opposite side of the body. That is, the left hemisphere deals with the right side of the body, and the right hemisphere the left side of the body. This fact explains why someone who has, for example, suffered a stroke in their left hemisphere may have difficulties in using their right arm and leg, sometimes to the extent of losing their use altogether. However, as we have seen, the two hemispheres are connected, and are in constant communication, so we should not imagine that we have two separate brains.

The lobes. We can see in Figure 4.2 that, apart from the two hemispheres, there are also different **lobes**. The lobes can be distinguished from each other by deep fissures, but although they are therefore anatomically distinct, the lobes are very closely pressed together. We do not need to go into much detail about what the lobes do, but we will briefly mention what functions they are particularly responsible for, although there is a great overlap between them. The temporal lobes deal with, amongst other things, the processing of **sound**, including music, speech etc. The frontal lobes deal with motor control (that is movement) which includes the ability to translate thought into

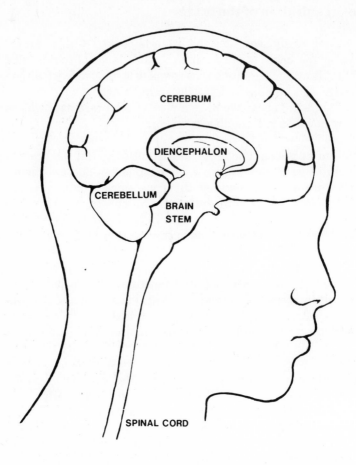

Figure 4.3 Cross-section of the human brain

speech. The frontal lobes are also involved in the complex area of **personality**. The parietal lobes are involved in receiving and interpreting sensory information, except for visual aspects, which are dealt with by the occipital lobes.

In very general terms, there are three forms of functioning involving the lobes, which occur in areas which, as we suggested above, overlap the boundaries of the lobes:

    (i)   The **sensory** areas: which deal with information from our senses;

   (ii) The **motor** areas: which deal with muscular movement; and

(iii) The **association** areas: which deal with the integration of complex intellectual and emotional processes.

Although we can say the functions tend to be **concentrated** in certain areas, the complex interconnections ensure that even the simplest experience involves the activity of different areas in the brain.

The areas we have looked at so far are those which are visible from the outside of the exposed brain. This outer 'layer' of the brain is known as the **cerebrum**. However there are deeper layers of the brain which we need to look at, and this we will do in the next section.

The deep structures of the brain. In Figure 4.3 across you can see a cross-section of the brain. The outer layer – the cerebrum – has already been discussed. As this is a cross-section the diagram shows one hemisphere of the cerebrum.

We can now see the deeper structures of the brain – the spinal cord, the brain stem, the diencephalon and the cerebellum. These deeper structures in a sense make up the 'old' brain. By this we mean that as human beings we have evolved from our more primitive animal ancestors, and our brains have likewise evolved. The outer layer is in this sense the 'new' brain, having evolved 'on top' of the old brain more recently, and it is in these newer parts that our specifically **human** attributes – intelligence, language and so on – are based. This gives us a clue to the functions of the older, deeper structures. They are specifically geared to the numerous essential 'life support' functions, which we take entirely for granted (until they go wrong that is!). A few examples of these life support functions are: the maintenance of breathing; the regulation of body temperature; the basic 'fight or flight' emotional and physical reaction; the regulation of hunger, thirst and satiation; the processing of basic environmental stimuli; waking and sleeping.

Memory and the hippocampus. An additional function which is crucial to survival is **memory**: any animal without memory would be hard pressed to survive for long, since they could not retain important information. In Figure 4.3 you can see the central parts of the brain known as the diencephalon. This contains a number of distinct structure, one of which is called the **hippocampus**, and it is the hippocampus which has been found to be crucial in terms of memory. Put very simply, what the hippocampus does is take in information from the senses, and, on the basis of how important that information is assessed to be, then transfers the information away to be processed and stored in other parts of the brain, or lets it fade away. In a way the hippocampus is a kind of filing system. It first of all decides whether information is worth keeping, and if it is, it decides on whether action is required, or whether it should be filed in long-term memory stores. These long-term memory stores will be in other parts of the brain. (However, it should not be supposed that each memory is stored in a specific part of the brain – this idea is far too simplistic. Instead there may be a highly complex integration of new and old information made in the association areas of the cerebrum.)

However, for our purposes here, it is sufficient to understand that damage to the hippocampus will have a major effect on memory. In the next section we will look at dementia in terms of the damage to the different parts of the brain, including the hippocampus and memory.

The organisation of the brain and dementia
Alzheimer's disease. People with dementia show a whole range of different symptoms. However the most distressing symptom, and one which affects every person with dementia, is the severe difficulty experienced in terms of short-term memory. The typical cause of this difficulty is damage sustained to the neurons comprising the hippocampus, and this damage is particularly the case in Alzheimer's disease. The effect of this damage is that **new** information is not processed well, if at all, and so new learning is very problematic. With mild to moderate degrees of dementia, the sufferer may still be able to learn new information but it will take him or her far longer. At more severe levels, no new learning will occur. It is very important to realise that the millions of memory traces laid down **before** the dementia will not be affected by hippocampal damage alone. Memories will be retained even at severe levels of dementia, and this explains why a person with dementia may forget things which happen minutes or seconds previously, and yet can have a lucid discussion about things that happened many years ago. In fact, in the example above, it may not be accurate to say that the person **forgot** what happened seconds previously, as the

information may not have been **registered** properly initially. In other words we cannot forget things which were never really received in the first place. In the later stages of Alzheimer's disease however, the areas of damage to neurons may occur all over the brain, and in this case there will be a number of other symptoms apart from memory loss. Damage to areas of the right hemisphere may lead to emotional difficulties – continual crying or laughter for example. Motor areas may be affected, making some movements difficult. All in all, as the disease progresses, there is likely to be increasing deterioration in a number of functions, although some may be left relatively unimpaired.

Multi-infarct dementia. The pattern of problems in MID may be very similar to that of Alzheimer's disease. However there may well be differences due to the different nature of the disease process, although memory will again be affected in all cases, as infarcts occur in the deeper structures already discussed. One difference is that Alzheimer's disease involves a slow and steady deterioration, whereas MID often involves abrupt changes in behaviour and mental functioning following infarcts which affect particular parts of the brain. This may be followed by some improvement as the brain makes a limited recovery from the trauma.

Because there are a number of factors that can affect the blood supply, the symptoms of a person with dementia may vary more, even on a day-to-day basis. This will be particularly the case in the early stages of the disease.

The location of the infarcts is again important in MID. For example, a person who is suffering problems with language – either speaking or understanding – is likely to have had infarcts in one of the lobes of the left hemisphere, possibly the temporal lobe, as this is involved in dealing with the processing of sound.

As MID progresses, the symptoms of a person may become very similar to someone with Alzeimer's disease, as both diseases involve increasing areas of damage within the brain.

Finally, we should mention that a significant number of patients may suffer both Alzheimer's disease **and** MID, and so may show features of both illness.

This long section on the organisation of the brain completes the main discussion of the brain and dementia. However, there are a number of other related areas that may be of interest to the reader, and so we will briefly cover these in the following sections.

Dementia and genetics

There has been a good deal of research looking at the possible inheritance of diseases relating to dementia. The general findings of this research suggest that there is an inherited risk factor; that is, someone whose parent(s) suffered from dementia has a slightly greater that average chance of suffering from dementia too. However, we must stress that this is only an increased **probability**, and that the association is not a very strong one, and so people who have relatives with dementia should **not** worry about developing it themselves.

Recent research has suggested that there is a specific chromosome abnormality in dementia sufferers, and this may prove helpful in future, especially in the early detection of the disease.

Dementia and aluminium

Aluminium is one of a number of toxic metals which are known to damage the nervous system. It has been found in higher than average accumulations in the brains of people with Alzheimer's disease at autopsy, and this has led to research looking at the possibility that aluminium could cause dementia. The evidence suggest that **by itself** aluminium is unlikely to be a cause, since if it were, far more people would be affected as aluminium is so common in the environment. Also it is not found in higher accumulations in the brains of **all** those with Alzheimer's disease. Nevertheless, although nothing definite is known, aluminium could be a factor for some people: for example it may be that something may trigger off a susceptibility to the metal, which in turn may increase the chances of developing a dementia-type disease. Generally though, the significance of aluminium is not yet well understood.

Other diseases which cause dementia

We've seen that over 90 per cent of elderly people with dementia are suffering from either Alzheimer's disease or multi-infarct dementia, or a combination of the two. However there are other much rarer types, which we will very briefly describe below.

Pick's disease. This is a very rare condition which is marked by a generalised atrophy of the brain, with the frontal and temporal lobes particularly affected. Although the course of the disease is very similar to that of Alzheimer's disease, in the early stages a sufferer tends to show changes in character and intellect, rather than memory. There is some evidence that Pick's disease is inherited and affects females more than males, but its cause is as yet unknown.

Jakob-Creutzfeldt disease. Again this is a very rare condition, but it differs from the other forms of dementia in that it tends to run a very rapid course: three to nine months from onset to death in 50 per cent of cases. This compares to five to ten years and longer for other forms of dementia. In Jakob-Creutzfeldt disease the damage to the brain is very extensive, with the deeper structures of the brain being attacked as well as the cerebrum. We have seen that the deeper structures are involved in 'life support' functions, and this explains the increased speed of mortality in the disease.

It appears that this condition may be caused by an infectious agent, known as a 'slow virus', which can incubate in the body over a long period of time. This is an important discovery as it raises the possibility of other degenerative conditions, such as Alzheimer's disease having a related infectious basis.

Huntington's chorea. This disease is a condition where the cause is reasonably well-defined. Again it is very rare, but it is inherited in the most direct and simple way from generation to generation. It is marked by 'jerky' movements of the limbs of sufferers, followed over a period of years by a gradual deterioration in mental faculties, the frontal lobes in particular sustaining damage. The age of onset can vary from between twenty five and fifty years, by which time they may have children of their own who have a one in two chance of developing the disease themselves. A test to establish whether a family member has the disease is now available. However, the decision to take the test is a very difficult one, so advice and good information is essential.

Summary

1 Although there are a number of diseases which can cause dementia, the two principal causes are Alzheimer's disease and multi-infarct dementia, which between them account for more than 90 per cent of cases.

2 Alzheimer's disease involves a process, the cause of which is as yet not known, which leads to damage in the structure of neurons, in turn leading to areas of damaged neurons. The brain is organised so that different functions occur in different locations. Therefore the effects of damage depend on where it occurs. However, damage is generally sustained in the hippocampus, one of the deeper structures of the brain, and the fact that this structure is involved in memory explains why short-term memory is so profoundly affected in people with the disease. Long-term memory may not be affected until the late stages of the disease. The course of Alzheimer's disease involves the slow and steady deterioration of mental and then physical faculties. There is no cure as yet.

3 The process of multi-infarct dementia involves numbers of small 'strokes' or blockages which lead to the death of areas of neurons through oxygen starvation. The course of the illness may be more 'jumpy' than that of Alzheimer's disease, as the patient suffers the abrupt deaths of small areas of neurons, rather than steady damage. However, as both diseases progress, their effects become harder to distinguish as both involve the progressive damage to areas of the brain. As in Alzheimer's disease the **location** of these areas of damage in the brain is significant in terms of the symptoms caused. The causes of MID often lie in the cardiovascular system, and so treatment which slows (but cannot reverse) the process of damage is sometimes effective.

4 Some people show evidence of both Alzheimer's disease **and** MID.

5 Although aluminium is popularly believed to be implicated in dementia, its significance is not clear, and it is unlikely to be a sole causal factor.

6 There is some evidence for the significance of inheritance in dementia, although the probability is quite low.

7 There are other diseases which cause brain damage leading to dementia, and these are very rare.

5 Drugs and dementia

Introduction

Elderly people consume more medicines and tablets than any other group. This is because they are more likely to suffer chronic disease and doctors naturally want to prescribe drug treatments to relieve their symptoms. However, any consideration of how the elderly use prescribed medicines must take account of two problems:

1 Elderly people in general show a greater sensitivity to drugs, suffer more side-effects and have a tendency to accumulate drugs in their blood because their bodies are less efficient at expelling them.

2 It is also more likely that elderly people will be taking not one but several, even many different drugs at the same time. This is a problem because some drugs interact with each other in undesirable ways.

Because of these characteristics elderly people may experience drowsiness, confusion and all manner of other mental and physical problems which are caused by the drug treatment itself.

Some drugs and medicines most often prescribed for elderly dementia sufferers are particularly troublesome in this way. For example, tranquillisers, mood-modifying drugs (like those given for depression), sedatives and sleeping pills all have a capacity, if not very strictly monitored, to cause drug-induced symptoms in people with dementia in addition to the symptoms that arise directly from the disease. As ever there is a danger of such symptoms being interpreted as merely a sign of worsening of a disease rather than arising out of the very treatment given by doctors to control it.

Drugs and the elderly

Only doctors can prescribe drugs, but the use and especially the side effects of medications are of vital importance to all those who care for the elderly dementia sufferer. Because of the illness, an old person's grasp on reality or their ability to carry out certain tasks is very vulnerable to changes inside and outside their bodies. A minor illness or infection, such as a cold or flu, can affect such a person in quite a dramatic way by causing delirium (see Chapter 3). The same is true of the side-effects of drugs which in a fit person may only cause annoyance and minor inconvenience, but in a person with dementia can lead to a major change in behaviour and the onset of new and distressing symptoms. The basic rule is **when such a person rapidly deteriorates in their behaviour or ability to think, suspect an illness or a reaction to drugs.**

This knowledge is important because sometimes the medicines given to elderly people are not as properly supervised as they should be. Elderly patients may be given repeat prescriptions from their general practitioner over many years without regular checks. A doctor may, in good faith, want to treat an illness but may be too enthusiastic in his or her treatment. For example, a doctor may wish to treat high blood pressure in an old person but gives the tablets initially at too high a dose. This may lead to problems of dizziness, fainting and falling in the patient and, as these side-effects develop, the doctor may give other drugs to **counteract** their effects, Now the elderly person is on two drugs instead of one and complications are more likely. Doctors may not be fully aware of drugs that an old person may already be taking at home because of tablets given piecemeal in the past without regular review. Elderly people – especially those with memory problems – cannot always remember what to take or when, or what they have already taken. Tablets can have been in the house for months or years and 'gone off'. Tablets may be taken irregularly or in 'fits and starts' which can be very dangerous. Finally there is the danger of deliberate or accidental over-dosage. Drug treatments can be a source of help to elderly people and their carers in controlling some of the symptoms of dementia but it must not be forgotten that they are also a source of danger and that precautions are necessary in order for them to be used safely. This calls for careful monitoring of the effect of drugs by the doctor and close supervision by the carer of access and safety.

Doctors and psychiatrists vary in their detailed knowledge of the effects of various drugs on elderly people. Prescribing medicines for physical disease is relatively straightforward compared to prescribing to control problems like restlessness, screaming, agitation and behaviour problems. Tablets, potions and medicines are seen by many of us as the only 'proper' treatment and also as an 'easy' way through difficult emotional and behaviour problems. Tablets are concrete things we can see and touch and put in our mouths. Taking or giving a tablet seems so simple in comparison with alternative ways of tackling a difficult behaviour problem (see Chapter 6). Drugs are quick and immediate and make us feel that **something definite** has been done to help. It may be a kind of relief or assurance to know that tablets are there when times get rough. We must therefore have sympathy for general practitioners who may be overwhelmed by such problems and requests for help. If there are few practical or support sources to call on, doctors can do little other than prescribe in an attempt to bring relief and satisfy the expectations of their patients. In particular, general practitioners are under pressure to treat the difficult or disturbing, like those who have dementia, in this way. Families differ one from another in their circumstances and in the degree to which they can **tolerate** difficult or troublesome behaviour. The same is true of staff in different homes and residential facilities for the old. In this regard, the **morale** of carers and staff is the important factor which in turn depends on how isolated they feel, what practical support they can turn to and what other pressures and commitments they have. Certainly surveys of hospital wards and old people's homes where many dementia sufferers live show a sizeable proportion on tranquillisers and sedatives. But such drugs are potentially hazardous because in an old person with dementia there is a small margin between a dose that helps a particular symptom and a dose which cause further symptoms.

Why are elderly people more sensitive to drugs? This is not yet fully understood but it is known that in older people it takes longer for medicines to be absorbed in the gut. The ability of the liver to break down (metabolise) drugs also decreases with age and drugs are not cleared from the body by the kidneys as efficiently as in the past. The result of these biological changes is that medicines can have a far more potent effect and remain in the body longer. Concentrations of medicines can therefore build up in the blood of an elderly person over a period of time leading to a kind of 'overdose'. In this way, a person can be reduced to a drugged 'zombie-like' condition and will remain so until the medicines in his blood have been reduced. Of course, the presence of a physical disease of the body like dementia means that an elderly person is even less able to cope with such drug effects.

How do drugs differ?

The potency or strength of any drug and the likelihood of its causing side-effects depends on the type and dose, how it has been taken as well as on the general health and condition of the person taking it. In general drugs can be taken by mouth (orally), injected directly into the vein (intravenously) or injected directly into muscle (intramuscularly). Most drugs taken orally in the form of tablets must first be absorbed in the stomach and take about half an hour to get into the bloodstream. Intravenous injection puts the drug directly into the blood and its effects are immediate. Injecting a drug into muscle causes the drug to become effective almost as quickly. In general, the longer it takes for a drug to become effective in the body, the longer it remains in the system. On the other hand the quicker the drug takes effect, the faster it is cleared from the system. Drugs also differ from one another in the length of time they stay in the body. This is sometimes referred to as a drug's 'half-life', that is, the time required for half the amount of the drug to be broken down or cleared from the body. This can vary from hours to days.

Drugs and dementia

In the remainder of this chapter we will discuss some of the drugs likely to be prescribed for elderly people with dementia. These are mostly drugs which act directly on the brain and central nervous system (tranquillisers, sedatives and the like) and which are given to control some of the more distressing symptoms of the disease. We will also mention some other classes of drugs which are prescribed for other conditions more common in old age (cardiovascular illness, Parkinson's disease and arthritis) but which can also produce behaviour disturbance as a side effect. Finally, we will draw attention to some possible **inter-**

actions between those drugs and popular non-prescribed medicines bought over the counter.

The three main types of drugs which act on the central nervous system are shown in Figure 5.1. They are the minor tranquillisers (sometimes called sedatives or benzodiazepines), major tranquillisers (also known as phenothiazines) and antidepressants (mainly tricyclics or MAOIs). Figure 5.1 also gives a brief description of what they are prescribed for and their main side effects. Every drug has two names and these are also given for each drug. A drug's chemical name is its basic or general name by which the drug is known. Its trade name is simply the brand or title given to the drug by the company which produces it. Most ordinary people know drugs by their trade name as this is the one that appears in newspapers and advertisements. For example 'Diazepam' and 'Valium' are the same drug. There is no difference between them except that 'Valium' is easier to say and probably more expensive.

The minor tranquillisers (the Benzodiazepines). These drugs have been available for thirty years and there are many different types. The most commonly prescribed for the elderly are listed in Figure 5.1. They reduce anxiety and arousal, agitation, and restlessness. They relax the muscles and are used as sleeping pills. They have largely replaced traditional sleeping pills like barbiturates which were extremely addictive. However, there are potential problems in the use of these drugs particularly for the elderly:

(a) They have a number of **side-effects** including drowsiness, slurred speech, weakness, confusion and possible memory impairment.

(b) Elderly people may become **dependent** on these drugs, that is, psychologically or physically **addicted** to them.

(c) **Tolerance** for a drug may develop which means that higher doses may become necessary to produce the same effect.

(d) **Withdrawal symptoms** when the drug is withdrawn or reduced can be severe. During withdrawal anxiety may be heightened and sleeplessness increased. This is because some benzodiazepines have a long half-life (that is, a long duration of action) and will remain in the body for several weeks. Sudden withdrawal should be avoided and a doctor's advice sought on how best to reduce the drug.

(e) Some minor tranquillisers, such as Mogadon and Valium, when used as **sleeping pills** and taken at night can cause a drowsy,

Class	Chemical name	Trade name	Prescribed for	Possible side-effects
Minor tranquillisers ('Sedatives')	Diazepam Oxazepam Lorazepam Nitrazepam Chlordiaze-poxide	Valium Serenid Ativan Mogadon Librium	Anxiety, agitation, bodily discomfort hallucinations	Drowsiness, confusion, disorientation Agitation may follow withdrawal
Major tranquillisers ('Neuroleptics')	Chlorpro-maxine Promozine Fluphenazine Trifluo-perazine Thioridazine Haloperidol Droperidol Flupenthixol	Largactil Sparine Modecate Stelazine Melleril Serenace Depixol	Aggression, agitation, hostility, delusions, hallucinations	Drowsiness, rigidity, tremor, salivation shuffling gait, slurred speech, restlessness, rashes, constipation
Anti-depressants (Tricyclics)	Amitriptyline Doxepin Trimipramine Lofepramine Mianserin	Tryptizol Sinequan Surmontil Gamanil Bolvidon	Depression, sleeplessness, poor appetite, self-neglect, slowness, hypochondira	Dizziness, urinary difficulty in urinating (getting started), dry mouth, constipation, sleeplessness, confusion
Anti-depressants (M.A.O.I.s)	Phenalzine Tranylcypra-mine	Nardil Parnate	-ditto-	-ditto- hypertensive crisis if combined with certain foods

Figure 5.1 Drugs prescribed for dementia

drugged state during the day. This is because of their prolonged action in the body. Getting the dosage and timing of sleeping pills right can be difficult and may need to be adjusted under medical supervision.

Tranquillisers can be effective in helping the elderly person with dementia. They do not cure any aspect of the disease but can tip the balance between the illness and their carer's ability to cope in a direction favourable to the old person and their family. However, because of the above problems the drugs have to be administered with great care. If possible, alternative methods to drugs should be used to reduce an elderly person's anxiety or help them to sleep. Often because of an early resort to tranquillisers simple alternative strategies are not considered. For example soothing, reassuring and talking to an agitated elderly person should be the initial response from carers. An extra blanket, a warm drink, physical contact, a bath, can all be helpful in calming and inducing sleep in such a person. In institutions like homes and hospitals for the elderly, there are several useful strategies to promote sleep without resorting to drugs: reducing the amount of noise and disturbance at night, giving more privacy by drawing screens around the bed, finding out from relatives what the old person's sleeping patterns were at home, addressing the issue of whether sleeping pills are given for the convenience of staff rather than the convenience of the patient and, finally, trying to prevent the elderly person sleeping during the day by activity and stimulation.

The major tranquillisers (the neuroleptics). The 'major' tranquillisers are so called both because they differ chemically from the benzodiazepines and because they are used to control more severe behaviour disturbance: extreme agitation, hallucinations and deluded ideas. They are also used in smaller doses for the day and night sedation of elderly people. Again the most commonly used drugs of this type are listed in Figure 5.1, but there are many others. The major tranquillisers are usually given in tablet form, but, because of the reluctance of many disturbed patients to take drugs, injectable versions of the drugs have been developed that need to be given on a weekly to monthly basis (Modecate and Depixol). Such injections would usually be given by a GP or community nurse. There is a lot of variation in the amount of dosage required to achieve the same level of sedation from person to person. Changes in the elderly person's state, which may include tolerance to the effects of the drug, may develop leading to increased dosage over time. But in general, the drugs are likely to be effective in elderly people at much lower doses. The major tranquillisers are quite powerful drugs and have a number of problems associated with their use.

(i) They can produce very **distressing side-effects**. These include shaking and tremor, repetitive movements of the limbs and especially of the mouth and tongue, a shuffling walk perhaps with a strong urge to move around. Elderly people also experience dizziness due to lowered blood pressure and loss of heat (hypothermia). Skin rashes and blotches, a parched mouth and constipation are further side effects.

(ii) Elderly people seem to be particularly at risk of developing **irreversible** side-effects. Some elderly people can be left with involuntary movements of their body even after the drugs have been stopped. This is a condition known as 'Tardive dyskinesia'.

(iii) **Other drugs** are frequently used to moderate the side effects of major tranquillisers. For example, the shaking and tremor and movement is quite similar to symptoms of Parkinson's disease. Therefore, anti-Parkinson's drugs are given to counteract these side effects. However, anti-Parkinson's drugs may themselves cause problems (see Figure 5.2). For example, they can actually make the symptoms of Tardive dyskinesia worse or they can affect the thinking of the patient as the following case illustrates.

Mrs Archer was seventy-two years of age. She lived alone in a one-bedroom flat and had moved there three years previously following the death of her husband. She had no children but was supported by a long-time friend who called regularly. Mrs Archer was admitted to the local general hospital after having taken an aspirin overdose and seen by a psychiatrist. She was found to be 'moderately demented' and suffering from a delusion that she was being persecuted by neighbours.

She was discharged on a major tranquilliser called Flupenthixol (Depixol) which was given by injection on a regular basis by a community nurse. In the next six months Mrs Archer was admitted again to hospital on no less than four occasions following falls. She had developed a degree of constant restlessness and agitation which was attributed to 'anxiety'. She also experienced dribbling from the mouth and a tremor which were recognised as being a side effect of the first drug, Depixol. The Depixol was withdrawn and replaced by a drug called Stelazine which is also a major tranquilliser and acts in much the same way but it is taken orally by the patient. She was also given another drug to counteract the side effects. That drug was Madopar, often given to patients with Parkinson's disease.

After discharge from hospital within a month Mrs Archer's condition deteriorated. She was becoming unable to care for herself and was hallucinating. She could hear neighbours talking about her and trying to get in. She took to her bed, became incontinent and extremely dirty. Neighbours, friend and community workers felt that she was incapable of looking after herself or co-operating with others. They pressed for some kind of hospital or residential care.

At this point, Mrs Archer's drugs were thoroughly reviewed in her home. In addition to Stelazine and Madopar she was also found to have an old supply of a sleeping tablet called Heminevrin which is a sedative often given to those undergoing alcohol withdrawal. It was felt that Mrs Archer's trembling and restlessness were a side-effect of Stelazine and that the worsening of her mental state was a side effect of the Madopar which had been given to control the side effects of Stelazine. All drugs were withdrawn.

The improvement in Mrs Archer's mental condition and behaviour was quite remarkable in the following two week period. There was no longer any question that she was suffering from dementia. She became continent once again, dressed herself and was able to engage in conversation. Her physical appearance improved and she was much more alert. Her ideas of persecution disappeared. Her real problems remained – the loss of her husband and loneliness. But for two years it was believed she had a major mental illness or dementia. Her symptoms were largely due to drug side-effects.

In Mrs Archer's case we see a number of problems:

(a) A drug effect causing restlessness and trembling may be misjudged as a sign of anxiety.
(b) Further drugs are prescribed all the while which only complicate the problem.
(c) Tremors, body rigidity and involuntary movements are common side-effects of powerful (major) tranquillisers.
(d) Sudden occurrence of such problems must be thoroughly investigated.
(e) Drug effects can lead to mistakes in diagnosis and irreversible effects. (Mrs Archer was seriously considered for long-term institutional care.)

The major tranquillisers or phenothiazines are powerful drugs often used in the treatment of mental illness such as schizophrenia. They are used for dementia sufferers as a sedative and as a means of controlling agitation, aggression, violence and other severe behaviour problems. Because of their considerable side-effects and complications they should be used only as a last resort. However some of these drugs are quite commonly prescribed for the elderly (particularly Melleril). Any elderly person showing symptoms like those mentioned above after starting on a major tranquilliser should be seen by their doctor to ascertain whether their symptoms are drug-induced.

Anti-depressants. These drugs described in Figure 5.1 come in two different types: mainly tricyclics and M.A.O.I.s (which stands for Monoamine oxydose inhibitor). They are different

Class	Chemical name	Trade name	Prescribed for	Possible side-effects
Anti-hyper tensives and diuretics	Indoramin Methyldopa Prazosin Amiloride Frusemide Cyclopenthi-azole	Baratol Aldomet Hypovase Midamor Navidrex	High blood heart failure, swellings	Disturbed thinking, constipation, lethargy, depression, headaches, disturbed behaviour, urinary incontinence (sudden urge), confusion)
Anti-arrhyth-mics	Digozin Verapamil Tocainide	Lanoxin Cordilox Tonocard	Irregularities in heart rate	Headaches, weakness, loss of appetite, dizziness, disturbed behaviour, rashes
Anti-Parkinson's	Orphenadrine Procydidine Levodopa	Disipal Kemadrin Madopar Sinemet	Symptoms of Parkinson's disease, shaking, tremor etc. and for symptoms arising as side-effects of major tranquillisers	Hallucinations, confusions, nighmares, disorientation
Anti-arthritics	Aspirin Indomethacin Chloroquine		Arthritis (swelling, faint pains, stiffness	Excitement, arthritics emotional disturbance
Gastro-intestinal	Atropine Metoclopramide Carbenoxolone	Maxolon Biogastrone	Acidity, upset, gas	Confusion

Figure 5.2 Drugs prescribed for other illnesses

drugs and are very rarely given together as they don't mix well, but each has the effect of raising the mood of a depressed person. Such drugs are not as commonly used in dementia as the previous drugs we have considered. However, they are some-times used in the early stages of the disease when a patient may be aware of their mental decline and become depressed as a result. They are also used to treat a special kind of depression which at first sight has symptoms indistinguishable from those of dementia.

Anti-depressants raise the mood of a depressed person but take two to three weeks to have any effect. A small dose of the drug is given first and built up over a period of time. The drugs are often successful in raising mood but the course of treatment is long and should be continually reviewed for at least six months.

Unfortunately anti-depressants may also have some unpleasant side-effects including dry mouth, constipation, blurred vision, dizziness, sleepiness and confusion. Tricyclic anti-depressants are very dangerous in overdose so the supply of tablets must be carefully supervised. Often doctors will not give more than a week's supply at a time. The onset or worsening of confusion that coincides with the elderly person taking such drugs should always warrant referral to a doctor as this may show an over-concentration of the drug with perhaps more serious consequences to follow.

Mr Cook was an 82-year-old partially-sighted man living in sheltered accommodation with his wife. Over a period of several weeks Mrs Cook called her husband's G.P. to say he was going senile, couldn't make sense, was crying a lot and had become very lazy. He was losing weight and couldn't sleep at night.

Mr and Mrs Cook had been married for fifty years but there had been difficulties in their relationship with Mr Cook being overly dependent on his wife and Mrs Cook being negative in her attitude towards him. The G.P. felt that Mr Cook was depressed and prescribed a tricyclic anti-depressant called Gamanil. In addition day care was arranged for both of them at a nearby centre run by the social services.

The couple attended the day centre three times a week, but staff became concerned about Mr Cook's condition. He was very inactive and difficult to motivate. He spoke only when spoken to and often his speech was nonsensical. Sometimes he would seem very confused and at other times his thinking seemed more rational. As time went on staff found him increasingly drowsy and he would sleep for long periods at the centre. He would occasionally complain of giddiness and had a number of falls.

His wife, Mrs Cook, was physically disabled and confined to a wheelchair. She was an active person and very much appreciated the attention and interest of others. Her account of her husband was that he had lost his ability to do things and that he was aggressive and awkward. Nevertheless his confusion and 'senility' added to the attention she received from others in the centre. The worsening of Mr Cook's condition suggested a drug effect. Enquiries were made with Mrs Cook's daughter who confirmed that her mother was giving the Gamanil at above the required dose in order to 'keep him quiet'.

C

The drug was stopped at once and over a period of weeks, Mr Cook's drowsiness, sleeping and falling subsided. His mental state became more stable but some confusion remained. Subsequently the anti-depressant was given again this time administered by the Warden in his sheltered flat. In time he became more responsive and active in the centre but his ability to think clearly did not improve. Most likely this man had an early dementia which had been worsened by a depressed mood and emotional problems brought on by long-term marital strife. Mr Cook's case illustrated the following points:

1. Sometimes depression and dementia can be present at the same time and can be difficult to distinguish.

2. Anti-depressants can cause confusion and actually be dangerous if not administered properly.

3. Sleepiness, dizziness and falling which develop around the time a drug is introduced should be suspected as being drug-related.

4. When given properly and in the right dosage anti-depressants are often of benefit to a depressed elderly person by raising their spirits. However, they will not affect a dementia in such a person.

M.A.O.I. anti-depressants are different from tricyclics such as Gamanil. They have all the side-effects of tricyclics (see Figure 5.1) but in addition if they are mixed with certain other drugs or foods they have the potential to raise blood pressure to a dangerous level. For this reason they are used much less often than tricyclics; usually as a second line of treatment when tricyclics have failed. They are sometimes prescribed for people with unusual depressions. Other medicines and drugs whether prescribed or bought over the counter **should not** be taken with M.A.O.I.s. Your doctor should leave a card indicating certain foods and drink which should also be avoided.

Summary

1 Drugs which act directly on the brain and central nervous system are the most commonly prescribed drugs for dementia sufferers. We have discussed the three main types of these drugs (minor and major tranquillisers and anti-depressants) and their possible side effects.

2 Such drugs can be of benefit to the dementia sufferer and their family but elderly people are very sensitive to such drugs and

therefore they must be very carefully prescribed and monitored.

3 Whenever possible alternative methods of dealing with a problem (company, taking out, stimulation, day care) should be tried before resorting to drugs.

4 None of the drugs we have described has any impact on the disease itself. Their use is as a means of controlling symptoms.

Other types of drugs

So far we have considered only those prescribed drugs which might be used in an attempt to relieve some of the symptoms of dementia. Elderly people may also have other medical problems, which may be linked to their dementia or independent of it, but which require drug treatment. Figure 5.2 shows classes of drugs given for other illnesses which can produce disturbed behaviour as a side effect. These include drugs which act on the cardiovascular system, such as high blood pressure reducers, 'water pills', blood thinners and heart medicines. Those suffering from 'Multi-infarct dementia' (see Chapter 4) are quite likely to be receiving such drugs as their dementia arises directly out of cardiovascular disease. Drugs given to treat Parkinson's disease can cause thinking to become disordered and certain medicines given for arthritis can have the same effect. All a carer or concerned member of staff can do is to be aware that such side effects do exist and to find out as much as possible about the drugs that their elderly person is taking.

Alcohol and 'Cold Remedies'. In nearly all cases alcohol and drugs do not mix well. An occasional drink can be very good therapy for an elderly person, even one with dementia. However, alcohol can enhance the effects of certain drugs such as the benzodiazepines causing excessive drowsiness. In fact alcohol should not be mixed with any of the drugs mentioned in this chapter. Attention needs to be kept on medicines bought over the counter from a chemist as these too can mix badly with tranquillising drugs. Even a drug like Aspirin can cause sickness, vertigo, confusion and psychiatric disturbances in an elderly person if it is not taken properly. There are a large number of possible bad interactions between different drugs but it is enough to know that they exist and to seek suitable advice if in doubt.

General guidelines and summary

1 **Few dosages**
Usually an elderly person will require only about one third to a half of the dosage given to a younger person. Due to biological changes and general health drugs stay in the system of an elderly person to a greater extent.

2 **Few drugs**
Be wary when an old person is taking lots of drugs. Check that they are all necessary. In general the rule should be the fewest drugs possible given the least number of times a day.

3 **Careful supervision**
Check that drugs are being taken properly at the prescribed dosage and at the right time. Ensure that tablets are not taken in 'fits and starts'. Store tablets in a safe place.

4 **Onset of symptoms**
Suspect any symptoms which start around the time of an introduction or change of tablets especially:
(i) drowsiness, agitation and sudden confusion (delirium).
(ii) shaking, tremor, involuntary and repetitive movements of the body.
(iii) constipation, dizziness and falling.
Such symptoms are likely to be drug-related.

5 **Old Drugs**
Elderly people are likely to have been on drugs for longer periods than young people. Suspect medicines which have been taken for a long time. What are they for? Are they still needed?

6 **Knowledge**
Find out about the side effects of the drugs an elderly person is on, how long they take to have effect, how long they stay in the system.

7 **Caution**
Some drugs are absolutely necessary for the treatment of disease and all drugs have side effects. **NEVER CHANGE THE DRUGS AN ELDERLY PERSON IS TAKING YOURSELF. ALWAYS TAKE ADVICE FROM A DOCTOR.** Remember, where drug treatment is necessary an elderly person may just have to be supported in coping with the side effects where these are unavoidable.

8 **ASK**
Knowledge of drug-caused effects does not call for night school or a degree in chemistry. Develop a good relationship with your doctor, pharmacist, geriatrician, nurse or psychiatrist – don't be afraid to ask and expect a proper reply.

6 The behavioural approach to dementia

Terms like 'senile', 'demented', 'organic' or 'confused' are often used generally to refer to any mental decline where the outlook seems to be hopeless. In fact, as we have seen in Chapter 3, there are many medical conditions that give rise to a confused state in an old person, not all of them irreversible. Even in conditions such as Alzheimer's disease, there is much individual variation in the symptoms shown and in the rate at which they develop. It is therefore quite wrong to assume that the characteristics that 'demented' or 'confused' people share are more important than the difference between them. Each sufferer is an individual in whom the particular expression of the disease will be unique.

This is important because those elderly people who have such terms applied to them are in danger of receiving services based on very low expectations of them. For example, in residential provision those with confusion or dementia are likely to end up in some of our least stimulating environments (long-stay hospital wards). In local authority homes for the elderly, being seen as confused can lead to significant losses of rights and privileges compared to so-called rational residents. In order to treat a person medically or help them in some other way, we must have a clear idea about what it is we are trying to treat or help. By themselves, terms like confusion or dementia may tell us everything we need to know in order to place a patient, but nothing that we need to know in order to help him or her.

From a psychologist's point of view labels such as 'demented', 'confused' and 'senile', which cover so much while telling so little, are of questionable value. It is much more helpful to describe the **behaviour** of the old person if we wish to influence it and to get away from terms which have taken on a pejorative value and from which little tangible action ensues.

Behaviour

We may speak of an elderly person's aggression, withdrawal or awkwardness and think that what we mean by these terms is self-evident. In practice, however, any two people would have a different idea of what was meant by them. They are our own inferences or hunches about what's going on inside someone, which we use to explain their behaviour. We don't have direct access to someone's aggression, withdrawal or awkwardness, we only **infer** it from what they **do**.

A person who is called withdrawn will actually be behaving in a certain way; for example, they may be avoiding eye contact, not responding to prompts, sitting alone in a corner, speaking only when spoken to. An aggressive person may be verbally abusing particularly people, throwing certain objects, hitting other residents. A wandering person may be pacing up and down near the front door, unable to sit for more than a few minutes or having to be found after repeatedly getting 'lost'. In all these cases, it is these more specific descriptions of what the person is actually doing that forms the basis of behavioural intervention.

Remember behaviour is action. It is something we can all see. It is therefore easier to agree on, easier to plan treatment for and easier to assess in order to see whether the treatment has worked.

The behavioural approach. The behavioural approach relates behaviours to specific objects, people or situations, and has been found to be useful with elderly people with a variety of diagnoses including Alzeimer's disease, M.I.D. and other disorders. It does not ignore or deny the reality of these diseases but simply says that many elderly people have a higher level of disability than is warranted by their health status. It is not a panacea nor a cure-all and it makes high demands on care-givers in terms of time and commitment.

This is because it focuses on the elderly person's needs as an individual (or it should do) rather than on 'easing the burden' for care-givers as its primary aim. We realise that carers and care workers are often under intolerable stress and this will be considered in the next chapter. However, too often the elderly person loses out when this equation is balanced against the interests of daughters, grandchildren, neighbours, community services or 'my other residents'.

Finally, the behavioural approach should not be viewed as a set of 'helpful hints and advice' but as a method for helping elderly people who now have **learning difficulties**. The approach is based on teaching principles that have been known for centuries and on more recent scientific research showing their effectiveness. The approach takes into account the diversity of factors operating on an individual person including but not limiting itself only to effects of the disease.

Deficit and excessive behaviours. The behavioural approach tries to understand the behaviour of an elderly person within an environmental and social context. It concentrates on what happens before, during and after behaviours of interest. Of course, not all distressing behaviours can be changed, or even need to be changed, but efforts should concentrate on those that cause most distress to the elderly person and their families.

Most behaviour problems can be thought of as occurring too · frequently or too little. Behaviours that occur too frequently are called 'excessive behaviours' and are easy to identify: wandering, repetitive questioning, screaming, incontinence are all examples of excessive behaviours. Behaviours which do not occur often enough are called 'deficit behaviours' and are a little more difficult to specify, especially in dementia where expectations of what an affected person can do may be low. But examples would be dressing, activity outside the house, getting out of bed, washing, shaving and so on.

Observation and recording. In any behavioural intervention a realistic outcome or goal is important. In effect this means strengthening any positive behaviours an elderly person has and also changing household or other conditions in order to compensate for physical limitations and memory problems. The approach assumes that, no matter how impaired a person is, they must have a strength, capacity or resource which can be used in trying to help them. The question to be decided is what should be different following intervention. This goal must be stated as specifically as possible. For example, 'Mrs Jones must learn to be aware of the dangers of using gas fires' is too vague. A more precise and useful version might be 'Mrs Jones will learn to turn the knob of the gas fire on and then light the filament'. Remember that the target behaviour must be observable and measurable when we are thinking about what Mrs Jones's behaviour could be like following interventions.

A problem like Mrs Jones's may be selected because it is of most concern to the family, or because it builds on something she is already doing or because she has someone there to help her with it. There may be two or three such problems being worked on simultaneously. However, each must be systematically observed and recorded. In fact, this kind of observation is a distinctive feature of the behavioural approach. We all make observations of others but usually these are not carried out in a systematic way. This means we must carefully observe the elderly person's current behaviour (that is, what he or she actually does at present) concerning our selected goal (in Mrs Jones's case turning on and lighting the gas fire). The first thing we do is to observe and write down how, when and why she turns on the gas so that we can see where the difficulties are. A record sheet like that shown in Figure 6.1 should be used for this.

This record will help us to answer a number of questions that we need to know before working out an intervention to help Mrs Jones. For example, does she actually try to light the gas? Is her memory about this better or worse at certain times or when certain people are present? Can she physically manage the knobs and matches? What prompts her to approach the fire? Does she show any signs of knowing that the gas is on, and so on. Where it is possible, as in this case because of the presence of a spouse to record every occurrence of the target behaviour (switching on the gas), then this should be done as this is the most accurate observation method. However, it is not always feasible to do this. Generally, it wouldn't be possible with target behaviours which are very frequent (such as repetitive questioning or shouting for help).

If it is not possible to observe and record every occurrence of a behaviour, then the next thing is to **sample** it in a systematic way. For example, an elderly person who constantly repeats the same questions could be observed for ten minutes every hour with the observer writing down how many times the same question was repeated during the ten minutes. This may seem like a lot of work, but in practice it is relatively simple. It helps us later on in deciding whether anything has changed and where we are either succeeding or failing. Note that the elderly person never fails, only our attempts to help them may fail – a distinction not to be forgotten in what follows.

Date _____

Time _____

Describe what person did _____

_____

_____

_____

_____

What was happening just before _____

_____

_____

_____

_____

What happened as a result _____

_____

_____

_____

_____

Other points _____

_____

_____

_____

_____

_____

Figure 6.1 Behaviour record sheet

Intervention

The primary aim of behavioural intervention is to reduce 'excessive behaviours' like shouting, verbal abuse, physical aggression, wandering and incontinence by strengthening positive, acceptable behaviours which are incompatible with these undesired activities. One way of increasing someone's functioning is by simply allowing them to do more. Many elderly people, and especially those diagnosed as having an organic disease or who are seen as 'confused', have many opportunities to do things removed from them by others 'taking over'. Expectations of them may be low, and this is often reinforced by an apparently hopeless diagnosis and by a vicious circle being created which produces dependency and despair (see Figure 6.2). For example, an elderly lady may be locked in her own house by concerned relatives because she lost her way on one occasion. A small accident at a cooker might similarly lead to complete disconnection of the supply. For busy staff in a residential home it may be quicker and more convenient to dress and 'toilet' residents rather than having to 're-do' elderly people who have attempted these activities for themselves, perhaps not entirely successfully. Besides, staff may feel that responsibility for the slightest accident may fall on them and therefore create a regime where hardly any 'risky' behaviour is allowed. Medical practitioners may inadvertently limit behavioural opportunities by prescribing tranquillisers, say, for verbal aggression, which have the effect of reducing all speech. The attitude taken to risk by family, carers and staff may be a major limitation to any intervention, behavioural and otherwise. Another way of helping the elderly person to do more is to increase those cues and prompts which naturally occur in the home environment. Prompts are simply reminders to the old person to carry out a particular activity. The most obvious example is simply asking someone to dress and then praising them for it. The more questions the old person is asked the more likely they are to speak. Prompting may help a memory disordered person to keep in mind various facts about themselves, their routine and their environment. In such a memory disordered person, continual prompting and reminding may serve as a bridge to keep them in touch with reality. Use of memory aids like signposts, different coloured doors for the toilet and other items such as a large clock, calendar, newspapers may

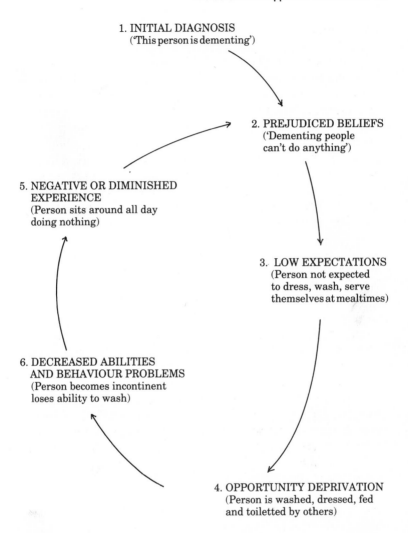

1. INITIAL DIAGNOSIS
('This person is dementing')

2. PREJUDICED BELIEFS
('Dementing people
can't do anything')

5. NEGATIVE OR DIMINISHED
EXPERIENCE
(Person sits around all day
doing nothing)

3. LOW EXPECTATIONS
(Person not expected
to dress, wash, serve
themselves at mealtimes)

6. DECREASED ABILITIES
AND BEHAVIOUR PROBLEMS
(Person becomes incontinent
loses ability to wash)

4. OPPORTUNITY DEPRIVATION
(Person is washed, dressed, fed
and toiletted by others)

Figure 6.2 The vicious circle affecting many elderly people

help. For someone with an incontinence problem, it makes sense that they should be within easy access of a toilet if they have any mobility problems.(More will be said about this under incontinence.) It is also important to ensure that the elderly person's problems are not due to sensory difficulties (very common in old age), that is, that their vision and hearing have been adequately tested and corrected.

It is a mistake to think that, because an old person may have lost their capacity to communicate adequately, they are no longer social beings. People with dementia are particularly vulnerable to loss of social contact and isolation, perhaps because the family are embarrassed or exhausted by behaviour problems or because of mobility problems, or because the old person fears leaving the house. It is important to use the community services that may be available in your area (see chapter 8) to promote social contact. Luncheon clubs, meals on wheels services, day care (statutory or voluntary), home help services and nursing care all bring the affected individual into contact with other people. Arranging such help can be a complex business but, in addition to providing increased opportunities for social contact, these services can also mean that the amount of care families need to provide can be reduced.

Reinforcement. Let us return here to our initial distinction between 'deficit' and 'excessive' behaviours. You will remember that the former are behaviours we would like to see more of, such as dressing, washing and self care, and the later are behaviours we would like to see less of, such as screaming, wandering and incontinence. For behaviours we would like to see increased, the main behavioural technique used is **reinforcement**. Reinforcement is a very important idea in the behavioural approach. It is any action which, when it follows a certain behaviour tends to make it more likely that particular behaviour will be repeated. Touch and attention are perhaps the most powerful reinforcers, although the degree to which these or other potential reinforcers influence behaviour will differ from one person to another. Other reinforcers may be discovered during the period of observation that may be equally as good. Of course, not all elderly people will respond to attention or touch. A good rule of thumb for finding out what **does** motivate them is to use an activity or behaviour which occurs often, to reinforce another behaviour which occurs rarely but which we would like to see increased. Thus special activities or behaviours enjoyed by the elderly person are specifically targeted to increase the frequency and duration of these desired behaviours. For example, for someone who loves to go out, an outing is used to reinforce their having washed themselves. For someone who likes cigarettes, smoking can be made dependent on their being out of bed.

Breaking down tasks. Mrs Jones's gas lighting problem is another example of a deficit behaviour (that is, she doesn't light the fire after she has turned it on often enough). Lighting a gas fire, like many other deficit behaviours such as dressing or washing, is in reality not one but a whole series of small tasks put together. Each component is a step towards the completion of the whole task. Mrs Jones's gas lighting task may involve the following steps:

(i) approaching the fire;
(ii) picking up a box of matches;
(iii) distinguishing which knob on the fire to switch on;
(iv) switching on the gas;
(v) taking a match from a box;
(vi) striking the match;
(vii) igniting the gas fire with match;
(viii) extinguishing the match; and
(ix) disposing of the match in an appropriate place.

The initial period of observation and recording should help us to locate where Mrs Jones's problem lies along this chain of events. For example, without being able to make a pincer grasp with thumb and forefinger, it is very difficult to strike a match. Similarly, without reasonably good mobility, it is difficult to bend down to a gas fire in order to light it. Identifying particular physical difficulties may then lead on to appropriate solutions (for example, the provision of a self-lighting fire and perhaps cooker, battery operated gas lighters, electric kettles and so on). On the other hand, observation may reveal physical co-ordination or memory disorder of such severity that the goal of enabling Mrs Jones to light the gas is no longer judged to be realistic. In such cases, radical action may well need to be taken to safeguard Mrs Jones and her neighbours (for example, gas disconnection together with an alternative supply of heating, food and drink). Attention would then shift to helping Mrs Jones with something else.

Let us suppose, however, that Mrs Jones has the physical capacity to independently use her fire and a memory of how to do it which is incomplete rather than absent. Having broken down the task into steps, we might see that sometimes she does attempt to light the gas. This behaviour would be reinforced by attention, praise, or similar, whenever it occurred, on the principle that any behaviour strongly reinforced is likely to occur more often. If, on the other hand, we were starting from scratch and trying to retrain Mrs Jones to use her fire because, say, she was refusing to switch it on in the middle of winter, we might start off by reinforcing her for just sitting in front of it with a blanket, and then, as this occurred more often, to change our criterion so that we would only reinforce her for something that was closer to our designed goal such as allowing someone else to light it for her. In this way, it might be possible to gradually shape Mrs Jones's behaviour towards our desired goal of using her fire in an appropriate way.

The most obvious way of training someone to do a task is to take each step in turn, making sure that they have learnt one step before going on to the next in the chain. This is the method most of us are familiar with for learning anything new. It is also the method used for constructing this chapter – with one section building on the previous one in what is hopefully a logical chain of development. This kind of learning is called **forward chaining**. Sometimes however, it makes sense and is better to start at the end of the chain of steps and work backwards. For example, let us take a man who has lost the ability to dress. The natural order of dressing for a man goes something like this; pants, vest, shirt, trousers, socks, shoes, pullover and coat or jacket. It would seem sensible in order to help such a man to identify the first step in his learning sequence as stepping into his pants with his carer finishing off the rest of his dressing. If this was successful the next task would be for him to pull his pants up, again with his carer finishing off the rest of his dressing and so on through the sequence: from pants to vest, from vest to shirt, from shirt to trousers and so on until the man had, in theory, learnt to fully dress himself up to and including putting on his jacket. However, it is more complete, more satisfying and more rewarding, for the carer to complete the dressing leaving the **last** step in the chain, that is the man learning to push his arms through the sleeves of his jacket and working back from the jacket to pullover, to socks, to shoes, to trousers and so on. This technique is known as **backward chaining** and is simply another way of helping someone to learn something. Its advantage over forward chaining is that on each occasion the disabled person completes or finishes off the whole task.

We have risked a little complexity with these examples in order to demonstrate some of the basic techniques in behavioural intervention. These could be applied to many other 'deficit' behaviours where our aim is to increase the frequency of those behaviours happening. You can see that a certain amount of detail is required in order to say who will be doing the helping, when and how often and how it is to be done. The important principles are the proper use of reinforcement, providing direct help to the elderly person, whether observing them, verbally prompting, demonstrating or physically guiding them, and then offering less help or fading out as they do more for themselves. Fading means offering less help as the training progresses. If the elderly person succeeds in a task (such as putting on an item of clothing) with a lot of verbal instruction from you, use a briefer reminder on the next occasion and see whether they are still successful. On a further occasion they might succeed with you just observing them silently, although you would have to set the scene by giving them a brief instruction such as 'Now I want you to put your coat on' or 'Turn the fire on', then you would remain silent while they tried. This process of fading out the extent of direct guidance given by the carer can be conceived as gradually coming down a flight of stairs (see figure 6.3).

Physical prompting means actually guiding the elderly person's limbs through the steps of the task. Demonstration then is physically showing how the task is done. Verbal instruction is taking the elderly person through the task. Silent observation is making no comment unless and until a mistake is made.

Unfortunately it is the case that many elderly people with dementia have great difficulty in learning and this is one of the distinctive features of dementia. There may therefore be the need for numerous training occasions and the realisation that fading out your help in the way suggested above may not be possible. However, it is better that a person continues to function at the maximum that their condition allows even if this requires lengthy verbal prompting and physical guidance by carers. The most basic principal to aim for is to give the minimum help

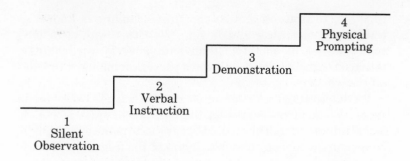

Figure 6.3 Fading out the extent of direct guidance

necessary and to give less help each time consistent with the successful completion of task by the elderly person.

The above techniques are valuable because they are sensitive to the differences between sufferers in their capacity to relearn or retain old skills; because many elderly people in the early stages of disease have varying mental incapacity and it is important to retain and encourage their functioning for as long as it is possible to do so; and finally, because a number of elderly people with characteristics resembling dementia may be wrongly diagnosed. When applied consistently, the kinds of behavioural techniques described have been shown to increase the likelihood of positive behaviour in elderly people, as well as providing additional stimulation for them.

Troublesome behaviour

Although the behavioural approach stresses the constructive by encouraging the search for behaviours to increase rather than others to decrease, it is recognised that many of the most troublesome and distressing behaviours seen in those with dementia are excessive behaviours (those that occur too frequently) such as wandering, screaming, incontinence and the like. It is these behaviours which are most likely to lead to a punishing response from carers, either out of desperation or with the idea that such behaviour requires very 'firm' handling. However, it must be said that punishment is hardly ever successful in reducing such behaviour, principally because these behaviours are rarely within the control of the elderly people exhibiting them. It should, therefore, be avoided at all costs.

It may still be possible to use reinforcements to decrease troublesome behaviour by choosing a behaviour to reinforce which is incompatible with it. For example, it is impossible for someone to be screaming and talking quietly at the same time. Your attention might, therefore, be used to reinforce the alternative behaviour of talking quietly whenever it occurs. In addition, you might be able to reduce the screaming by extinction; that is, by removing any attention which was tending to maintain the screaming. Screaming in an institutional setting like a hospital ward often attracts attention, even if it is angry attention from other people, which inadvertently reinforces it. Paying a person very little attention when she is screaming but lots of attention when she is talking quietly or knitting or whatever can have an effect.

Even with these difficult behaviours the behavioural approach would prompt us to think positively. For example, wandering or otherwise causing disturbances on the street can lead to one negative solution; that is, preventing an old person from going out. This too will have its drawbacks in that a person's reaction to confinement may result in further distressing behaviours developing.

Let's take some examples: a formerly very respectable elderly lady was accused of shoplifting, having walked out of a shop with a basketful of groceries. On observation, the problem seemed to be simply a failure of memory. A proposed solution was a simple verbal prompt. Shopkeepers who knew her well were asked to simply remind her, 'Don't forget to pay for your shopping Mrs Rider' as she passed them by. Not all the shopkeepers were prepared to do this and some simply barred her. Yet this lady continued to spend most of the day wandering around the shops. The local police were also informed so that any incident in a shop could be dealt with without fuss.

Another example is of a woman who turned up at the local post office every day to collect her pension and would become extremely abusive if she was refused. Again, simple failure of memory together with eager expectation of pension day, resulted in her feeling that every day was pay day. The initial solution was to use home help and family to prompt her as to what day it was but this had no effect. The second solution was to come to an arrangement with the post office so that part of her pension would be paid every day.

An elderly man was found lost on several occasions miles away from his home having travelled there by bus. Careful analysis showed that his problems coincided with the introduction of bus deregulation in the locality. The solution was a retraining approach to help this man identify the right bus together with a wrist band giving his identity and a number to call in the event of his getting lost in future.

All these interventions are expensive in terms of time, but this must be set against the expense of confinement. They also call for a certain amount of ingenuity in coming up with good interventions. The risks to a confused person outside are undoubtedly greater than for those with all their mental faculties. But how much greater, it is impossible to tell. It is an individual decision to be taken by those closest to the old person, if he or she is unable to express a view. What may be the best for family and professionals may not be the best for the elderly person. Decisions regarding risk are best shared either with other members of the family and/or professional workers.

Summary of stages in the behavioural approach

1 **Describe** the problem behaviour as precisely as you can, that is, what the elderly person **does.**

2 **Observe** it in a systematic way over a reasonable period (at least a week).

Record when it occurs, how often, what precedes it, makes it worse modifies it or interrupts it. Look for physical problems, difficulties in surroundings, signs of ill-health.

3 **Analyse** your observations making hunches or informed guesses about why the behaviour is occurring and then generate possible solutions. It is the quality of the initial observations that is all important in leading us to ingenious solutions to the problem.

Figures 6.4 to 6.7 contain four examples of problems described together with tentative hunches as to what may be causing the problem and some proposed solutions. Neither the possible causes nor the possible solutions are meant to be exhaustive but are merely illustrative of this, the most important stage of the behavioural approach.

Figure 6.4 Problem: sits in chair all day

POSSIBLE CAUSES (Informed guesses based on observations)	POSSIBLE SOLUTIONS
Depression.	Seek psychiatric treatment.
Not allowed to do things as may have an 'accident'.	Look again at attitudes to to 'risk' - discuss with family/professionals.
Lack of stimulation or inappropriate, demeaning activities provided (e.g. silly games, quizzes, etc.).	Introduce activities/ stimulation based on previous interests and experiences.
Physically unfit/unwell.	Medical examination programme of gradual exercise.

Figure 6.5 Problem: taking clothes off in public

POSSIBLE CAUSES (Informed guesses based on observations)	POSSIBLE SOLUTIONS (generated by analysis of possible causes)
Results in immediate physical contact.	Give more physical contact when dressed. Minimise contact when undressed.
Going to toilet in the wrong place.	Remove to toilet with minimum of fuss. Reminders signpost/colour code toilet and train.
Expression of sexual desire.	Ignore if possible perhaps combined with lots of reinforcement when dressed.

4 **Intervene** by setting a reachable goal and choose a simple, flexible, humane plan. Outline a strategy and inform others. The basis of this intervention will be one or more of the proposed solutions to a problem but the intervention strategy must be 'spelled out' in detail so that all those in contact with the elderly person act concertedly to implement the plan.

5 **Continue** your observations to see if there is any improve-

Figure 6.6 Problem: reversed sleep pattern

POSSIBLE CAUSES
(Informed guesses based on
observations)

POSSIBLE SOLUTIONS

Sleeping (cat naps) during
the day.

Wake up if found dosing
during the day.

Lack of sufficient physical
exercise/mental stimulation.

Take out, arrange more
activities especially physical
exercise like walking. Increase
visits/stimulation during day.

Patterns of light or dark.

Introduce clearer getting up and
going to bed times. Draw back
curtains during day, make sure
there is plenty of light.
Turn off lights at night.

Figure 6.7 Problem: refuses to undress

POSSIBLE CAUSES
(informed guesses based on
observation)

POSSIBLE SOLUTIONS

Dislike of cold.

Extra heating.

Clumsy manner of undresser.

Change carer. Suggest
milder handling.

Shame, embarrassment.

Introduce non-family carer.
Show no disapproval.
Minimise upset. Be matter
of fact.

Lack of co-ordination of limbs.

Give physical guidance when
undressing without doing it
for the person.

Doesn't know which clothes
are which.

Putting clothes out in
order. Physical/verbal
guidance

ment. Remember that failure is not the old person's fault but a
reflection on the particular strategy employed. If necessary, try
again.

Incontinence

Now let us turn to the problem of incontinence and look at what the behavioural approach may have to offer here. Incontinence is one of the most common disabilities in those suffering from dementia and is often the major reason for admission of such people to nursing homes, hospitals and local authority care. Mental alertness is a major factor in maintaining continence. Therefore, any disturbance in mental alertness may predispose an elderly person to developing such problems.

Incontinence is, of its very nature, very distressing to family, carers and the elderly person themselves who quite frequently will deny all knowledge of it or blame someone else for it or hide it or simply become unconscious to it. It is a taboo subject with a strong stigma attached. Such lack of control over the bladder or bowel signifies a baby's lack of control, reinforcing the stereotype of old age as a second childhood. Also, because the social rules of toileting are so strong, incontinence, despite being caused by mental or physical illness, may still be viewed as an antisocial act. What exactly is meant by incontinence? Most simply, and in terms of behaviour, we mean that a person is not wetting or soiling in an appropriate place. Incontinence is a complex problem and again it is important to specify the problem by taking a base line, that is, recording all wetting and independent toileting behaviours shown by the elderly person for, say, a week.

It is important not to forget that there are often physical and environmental causes of incontinence. The main factor in the development of incontinence in those with dementia will be the presence in varying degrees of uninhibited neurogenic bladder. This is the loss of neurons (See Chapter 4) in the brain leading to faulty control over a lower reflex (contraction of the bladder). The elderly person may get insufficient warning because of this and may show a pattern of being too late. It is also important to be aware of infections in the bladder or urine tract which are also common causes of incontinence. In fact, there are a whole range of localised changes which can cause urinary problems in an old person, including vaginitis, prolapse, pelvic floor insufficiency (in women) and enlarged prostate glands (in men). In all cases, the physical causes of incontinence must be thoroughly investigated by a doctor, even if the elderly person has a diagnosis of dementia, as many of these causes are treatable.

Detailed observations may reveal other potential causes. The buildings, furniture, decorations and people around an old person may limit what that person can do. For example, not being able to climb stairs to get to a toilet will cause incontinence. Toilets which are too distant or too awkward to get to will cause incontinence, either because people wet themselves on the way or because they stop even attempting to get to the toilet. An old person may require physical help but may be too embarrassed to ask. They would have to be tactfully approached. Poor eyesight or a poor sense of direction will cause similar problems and may be helped by large clear signs and most importantly by good lighting. The environment in the toilet is also important. Handrails may be needed for support, or the height of the toilet seat itself might require adjustment. Toileting an elderly person at regular intervals may be a help. Your behavioural observations should help you to assess when and how often they need to go to the toilet in order to remain dry. When this is done, you should try to teach them to go to the toilet at these times, even if there is no strong urge to do. A small reminder, or limited help at appropriate times, can be very effective in maintaining an elderly person's toileting behaviour.

The behavioural approach applied: an example. Let's take the following example of how the behavioural approach might be applied. Mrs Smith is seventy-five years old. She lives in a small flat in warden controlled accommodation and has done so for five years. She had started bed-wetting three years previously, during a period when she was in hospital briefly following a fall. The problem continued when she was discharged back to her flat. In fact, she soon became incontinent during the day. She was diagnosed as suffering from an organic illness of the brain (dementia). She was undoubtedly seriously impaired in her functioning and in her awareness of her surroundings. She sat most of the time staring into space. However, she knew and enjoyed the attention of the warden. For the warden, the incontinence was a very time consuming and stressful problem. Simple but careful recording was carried out on a daily chart, for a fortnight. The following is a fairly typical example of the daily chart on Mrs Smith's incontinence.

DATE	TIME	✓ WET ✗ DRY	WHAT HAPPENED	OTHER COMMENTS
15 August	8.00 a.m.	✓	Got her up, changed bedclothes, washed, toileted and dressed her in new underwear and clothes. Put her in chair, made her cup of tea and breakfast.	With her for half an hour. Told her I can't spend all this time. I have other residents.
	10.10 a.m.	✗	Popped in. Mrs Smith was sitting in her living room. She was dry. Left to get on with other things.	Took her to toilet - nothing happened.
	12.15 p.m.	✓	Came to bring her down to lunch. Wet again. Had to help her change underwear and pads. Late for lunch.	None
	2.00 p.m.	✓	Mrs Smith in communal lounge since lunch. Took her to toilet. Then I walked her back to her flat.	Told her off
	4.30 p.m.	✗	Checked Mrs Smith. She was dry.	Wouldn't go to the toilet
	6.00 p.m.	✗	Eating her dinner in dining room. Everything fine. Didn't speak to her.	
	8.15 p.m.	✗	Called on her. Took her to toilet. Brought her down to communal lounge for sing-song. She enjoyed it.	She used the toilet
	9.30 p.m.	✗	Helped her undress. Put her into bed.	Didn't stay long

Figure 6.8 Mrs Smith's daily incontinence chart

This chart tells us quite a lot about Mrs Smith's problem. Firstly, we can see that she is found to be wet on no less than three occasions on that day, and on other days sometimes more. Secondly, if she is to be found dry this is most likely to occur in the evening. We learn that if Mrs Smith is found wet, her warden changes her underclothes, washes her, dries her, dresses her and positions her back in her seat. If, on the other hand, she is found dry by the warden, nothing in particular happens. After having made her check the warden leaves the flat. The fact that Mrs Smith is sometimes found to be dry and that there is a pattern to this in that she is most likely to be found dry during evening checks suggests that there may be a behavioural component in her incontinence and that something must be happening in the evening to maintain her continence at this time, at least occasionally. This might have something to do with Mrs Smith's pattern of fluid intake throughout the day or the fact that on occasions the warden would bring her down to the day room for entertainment evenings from time to time.

It might be that the physical contact or the presence of the warden in the flat during the time that she washes and changes Mrs Smith is in some way a reinforcement to her. This is not so surprising if it is true that she has little contact with anyone else. Such a suggestion does not necessarily mean that Mrs Smith is consciously or deliberately wetting but simply that the conditions of her care might be making it more difficult for her to remain dry. The record demonstrates that the warden plays a very key role in Mrs Smith's life and that in some way her delivery of care to Mrs Smith is linked to her incontinence problems.

POSSIBLE CAUSES	POSSIBLE SOLUTIONS
Uncontrolled fluid intake.	Talk to district nurse about how and when to limit fluid intake
Lack of contact/stimulation.	Refer to day centre. Bring more people to see her and keep her company. Talk to family about more frequent visits
Inability to make her need for the toilet known to others.	Start system of regularly prompting and questioning her to help her realise when she requires the toilet
Warden's presence and attention while she clears up is reinforcing the problem	Reorganise warden's contact with her to a way likely to reinforce her for staying dry

Figure 6.9 Mrs Smith's urinary incontinence during the day

The guesses that we have made about the possible causes of Mrs Smith's incontinence problem might be summarised in the following way together with a possible solution for each of the hunches we have generated.

Because we have arrived at a list of potential solutions does not mean that all the proposed solutions should be acted on all at once. A judgement must be made on which would be most likely to have an impact, easiest to carry out and least intrusive to Mrs Smith. In this example it was decided to work on the last two on the list: helping the warden to start a system of regular prompts and changing the way the warden delivered her care to Mrs Smith. The goal chosen was that Mrs Smith should be dry during the day with the warden helping to toilet her on request.

Intervention. 1. The warden was to call on Mrs Smith as before at two hourly intervals.

2. The warden would check her for wetness and record. Mrs Smith would be asked if she was wet or dry and the warden would tell her whether she was right or wrong.

3. If she was dry, the warden would stay with her for a while, making it clear why she was doing so. She would say, for example, 'You're dry Mrs Smith; that's good. It makes my job easier. That means I can stay a while with you and talk.'

4. Mrs Smith would be asked whether she wanted to go to the toilet. 'Do you want to go to the toilet now? I can help you.' If Mrs Smith answers 'yes' or shows she wishes to go to the toilet in some other way, then the warden shows the same approval as in 3, by saying, for example, 'That's very good, it means I can stay with you longer'.

5. If Mrs Smith was wet on checking, then the warden would let her know: 'You're wet Mrs Smith. I'll clean you up but that means I cannot stay with you.' No further conversation would be offered. The warden would leave immediately on completion of her task.

6. Further notes on the programme were as follows:

There was to be no arguing, encouraging or criticising. If Mrs Smith was wet, the warden would follow instruction 5 to the letter. This was done matter of factly. The warden continued to keep a record of Mrs Smith's continence and the programme was reviewed every two weeks and changed as necessary or discontinued.

Comment. It is important to realise that the warden's 'matter of factness' and not staying with Mrs Smith if she was wet is not a punishment; it is simply a reversal of what was happening before. Now the warden's time and attention, which we assume is valued by Mrs Smith, is reinforcing her dryness and not her wetness. This is the central feature of this particular intervention. Furthermore, the warden's clear questioning and verbal prompts are aimed at helping Mrs Smith to learn to control her bladder more effectively. She is now getting clear information from the warden on how she is doing, that is whether on each occasion she had succeeded or failed. One final point is that an attempt was made, and always should be made when possible, to explain to the elderly person the nature and purpose of the intervention.

After some initial difficulties on the warden's part in putting the programme into action, Mrs Smith's wetness reduced from over three to four times a day to once or twice a day, and within a week she was dry throughout the day with two hourly checks. She remained incontinent however, at night. It is interesting that, as Mrs Smith improved, her warden became reluctant to spend as much time with her. This was despite the fact that she was spending only half the time with her that she was prior to intervention when she was having to be cleaned three to four times a day. Sometimes the expenditure of time given to promote independence can be viewed by carers as spoiling or giving in, whereas time spent in the relentless and unrewarding pursuit of demanding behaviour is seen as part of the job. Each elderly person requires preferential treatment and the behavioural approach helps us to understand some of the elderly person's needs. It should never be a means of control but one way of trying to improve an individual's quality of life.

Summary

The behavioural approach concentrates on observable, self-evident behaviour which we can directly see and agree on. It avoids vague, internal concepts, such as motivation or agitation, over which disagreement is highly likely. A behavioural description of confused behaviour puts the emphasis on **what** happens and **when** and is not as concerned with **why** a behaviour problem occurs. No assumptions need to be made about underlying cause (such as dementia). When behaviourally describing a problem, diagnosis and symptoms are largely redundant.

Behaviour is specifically pin-pointed and recorded in a systematic way. Special attention is paid to what precedes, modifies or interrupts a behaviour, together with physical limitations, daily routine and current health. Such information is examined with a view to setting a realistic and attainable goal. A simple and humane intervention plan is drawn up. Such a strategy must be evaluated carefully and all those involved with the elderly person must be informed, including the old person in question. Any strategy must be looked at again regularly and changed as necessary. Strategies may fail, but the old person never fails. Behavioural intervention is the systematic application of basic learning principles.

7 Stress in carers

In this chapter, we will look at the stress which can occur in a situation where someone – usually, but not always, a relative – is helping or caring for a confused person. Stress, like most frequently used words, is not as simple as it at first appears, and so we will look at the different aspects that make up stress later on. But first of all we will describe a situation in which a person who is looking after a relative experiences stress and strain.

John Thorpe is seventy-four years old. He suffered a major stroke seven years ago and since then he has suffered many small strokes (known as multi-infarct dementia), which have left him severely disabled. He can walk with a stick, but his short-term memory is badly affected. His attention span and ability to concentrate are likewise affected such that he can do few of the things he used to. He was an active gardener and had been involved in a number of local organisations, such as the social club related to the job from which he retired – senior engineer in the local works. His wife, Pam, describes him as having been a very confident, popular, though at times over-bearing man. Pam is quiet and gentle, and has been deeply affected by John's condition.

'He is such a different person now. He even looks different he has lost so much weight. We've always had a good marriage, and, though he was always 'the boss' when it came to major decisions, we used to share a lot of other things together. His assertiveness made up for my lack of confidence, though I think I helped him to be a bit more thoughtful as well – he could be quite overpowering at times! Although his first stroke left him badly paralysed, he did seem the same person "underneath" if you see what I mean, and he did manage to recover quite a bit. He then started to suffer lots of what the doctor called mini-strokes. She told me that sometimes they are so small that the person it happens to doesn't really notice. Each one does some damage though, and John steadily changed. He lost his thoughtfulness, and instead was left with this overbearing part of his personality. He'd get angry with me if I tried to help him dress, for example, and insisted on trying to do it himself, although he'd get so frustrated he'd end up almost tearing his clothes. My daughter, Lorraine, is married and lives nearby, and she and her husband used to come for Sunday lunch regularly. It became very difficult though because John would pick arguments with anyone, Bill my son-in-law in particular, and because he couldn't really argue properly because of his memory problem, he'd end up shouting, and being very rude at times. Bill didn't seem to understand how affected John is, so he argued back just as angrily. They've stopped coming Sundays now, although Lorraine comes to visit regularly, thank goodness. This rudeness is something I find very hard to take, as John was never that way inclined. He's called me some terrible things since this all started. When he shouts at me I often end up shouting back and we both get really upset. I feel so guilty afterwards because I know it's not really his fault, but I can't help it. When he first started shouting I just cried, but you can only cry so much. I have to admit once I got so upset that I slapped him, he would have tried to slap me back but he's so weak now. I've never felt so depressed and guilty as then.

'One of the worst things has been the loss of our friends. I've felt I couldn't "inflict" John on friends, so we've stopped visiting (it's difficult travelling as well as I don't drive our car and John of course can't anymore) and though a few close friends do visit, I feel very uncomfortable in case John flares up in a rage, which he has done at times. Perhaps it sounds bad but I suppose I feel ashamed of John. Remembering what he was like before makes me feel ashamed for him as well. I can tell friends and acquaintances feel very sorry for me, but somehow their pity only makes me feel worse. I really feel that quite a few people we used to be friendly with now avoid me. A community nurse comes and calls sometimes, and he tells me to be patient with John and try to help him to do things, but that's so easy to say, and so hard to do. People really don't realise what its like, day after day. In the past few years I've started suffering frequent headaches, and I feel tired and low a lot of the time. I find sleep difficult, especially as John is restless at night, and needs to be taken to the toilet often. I saw my G.P., but all she could give me was tranquillisers and sleeping tablets, which I've been on for more than a year now. Despite it all I'm determined to carry on looking after John. I couldn't bear to see him in a home, and I know he couldn't bear to be in one. After nearly forty years of marriage that would seem terrible. But as I said before, he does seem a different person now, though every now and again there are flashes of the old John. I could show you photographs of him before his problems and you wouldn't think he was the same person. I don't think anyone can possibly truly understand what it is like to be looking after someone who used to be so strong, but who is now so weak.'

Pam's story is based on a carer's real experience. Although it is only a brief story, it does give us a picture of the sort of stress faced by carers. As stress is such a general word, it will be useful to split it up in terms of the three different kinds of reactions that are experienced when a person is looking after a confused relative or friend. Firstly there is the psychological or emotional strain, secondly the physical strain, and thirdly the social strain. We will look at each in turn.

The psychological or emotional strain

The pain of seeing deterioration in the personality of someone with dementia is probably the strongest reaction that carers experience. Despite this, it is often the case that the pain experienced by carers is not acknowledged by others, even close friends and relatives. Perhaps the reason for this is the strength of the pain, which people may recognise but don't know how to cope with, and so stay away or avoid talking about the subject. We can see from Pam's story that she doesn't get a great deal of support in terms of having someone listen to her, except perhaps for her daughter, who is likely to be very involved as well.

Carers are often likely to feel frustrated and annoyed as activities like dressing and washing can become lengthy and irritating for both the carer and the elderly person. Another problem is that many carers are not just looking after one relative, but are trying to fulfil other roles as well. As we saw in Chapter 1, most carers tend to be female, and so are more likely to involve other caring roles such as being a wife and a mother, sometimes with little help from the men in the family who feel it is 'not their job' to do this kind of work. At its worst, this kind of problem can lead to actual violence towards elderly relatives. Pam once slapped John, but in some situations things can get far worse, as we've seen in recent years in the increasing awareness of 'Granny-bashing'. The term itself trivialises elderly people.

We do not speak of 'kiddy-bashing' but rather of 'child abuse', which almost suggests that violence towards children is taken more seriously.

The psychological strain also shows itself in terms of depression, and again with Pam we can see that she experiences continual 'low' feelings. Many carers are also likely to be preoccupied with problems, worrying constantly, seldom able to 'switch off'. This leads to the second stress.

The physical strain

This involves two sorts of stress: firstly, the physical strain of looking after someone who may need a lot of bodily help; and secondly, the strain the carer experiences in terms of his or her bodily reactions. We will look at this second type in more detail, as it is less obvious, though often more significant. Pam's physical reaction involved physical (muscular) tension, leading to what are almost certainly tension headaches, and related to this a continuous feeling of tiredness, again partly due to muscular tension. We all need to switch off and relax particularly if we experience stress at work or at home. As carers are often spending large amounts of each day in face-to-face contact with an elderly person who is confused, they are very likely to develop a significant level of physical tension, as well as the emotional reactions already mentioned. This sort of physical tension can slowly build up over a number of weeks, months, or even years, and the person experiencing tension in this way may not notice anything especially wrong. However, that person will experience 'chronic' symptoms like tiredness, nervousness and irritability, inability to relax. At higher levels of tension, the carers may experience symptoms such as palpitations, anxiety (panic) attacks and dizzy feelings, each of which suggests that the level of physical tension is quite high. This sort of strain may affect other areas of the carer's life, such as the following.

The social strain

One noticeable feature of Pam's life is that her social life had become very badly affected following John's illness. Just as it is very hard for the husband or wife to adjust to their partner's deteriorated condition, so friends and acquaintances won't know how to deal with this new situation. The passage below is a description by Alex, a long-time friend of John's, of his reaction to John's illness.

'I've known John for thirty years. We worked together at the factory, and got to know each other very well. With our wives we've been a foursome for a long time. After John's first stroke it was difficult, but you could see him recovering and eventually you could have a good chat with him, he was always a good talker. However after all the other strokes he really seemed different. I've got to admit that I did not know what to say to him. I've never had any dealings with confused people, and, well, I just felt a bit lost. Mavis, my wife, felt the same too, and we both felt guilty that we couldn't give Pam more support. In fact Pam seemed to be coping fine, and in truth she doesn't seem too comfortable when we are there, so we don't call round so much now. I do wish we could be of more help though.'

Alex's reaction is probably typical of many people who have seen their friends become confused. Perhaps the most significant feeling is that of **awkwardness,** not knowing how to relate to a confused person, especially if it is someone you know well. The only way to overcome this awkwardness is of course to spend time with the person, learning how to converse with him or her, to find those areas in which confusion is minimal. We will look at this later, but from the above account it can be seen that there is a vicious circle in operation. Pam feels guilty about 'imposing' John on old friends and is uncomfortable when they are around in case John becomes difficult. Friends sense this discomfort, and also find it difficult to know how to talk to John. They don't have a 'feel' for his difficulties, and are uncertain as to his remaining abilities. So they tend to reduce their contact, especially as Pam **appears** to be coping well – as is often the case with carers. The result for many carers is that they become socially isolated: friends, neighbours and family may still call, but they don't get the closeness they had before, often because the person they care for is in when people call, and conversation centres around how he or she is, not on the carer. This isolation can lead to carers feeling that no one cares for them, leading to resentment and perhaps hostility, and this will further 'push away' people who visit.

To summarise

1 *The psychological strain* involves:
   a) The **pain** of seeing someone you are close to become enfeebled.
   b) Feelings of helplessness, depression and sometimes anxiety.
2 *The physical strain* involves:
   a) The straightforward exhaustion due to the physical burden.
   b) The (often unnoticed) build-up of physical (muscular) tension, leading to headaches, tiredness, insomnia and other problems.
3 *The social strain* involves:
   a) The carer feeling uncomfortable or nervous when people visit.
   b) Friends, neighbours and relatives may have no experience in talking to confused people, and so are very awkward and spend little time in learning **how** to relate to confusion.
   c) The carer consequently becomes socially isolated. Even if he or she has visitors, they may well only provide superficial social contact. Resentment and hostility can sometimes build up.

Coping with stress

Often the last thing carers want is advice. However most of the suggestions below come from carers themselves, as we wished to bring their experiences together to give an idea of possible approaches to difficulties that often seem unsurmountable. We will use the three sorts of stress outlined above as a guide to these possible approaches.

The psychological/emotional strain

The pain of caring. The pain of looking after a relative has been looked at briefly. One of the principal difficulties is not being able to share or discuss this pain and keeping it bottled up. Organisations such as the Alzheimer's Disease Society (whose address appears at the end of this book) are of course very important in bringing together people to share their experience, but in the example below the Society did not have a branch in the town where the carer lived, and, unusually there were no other carers' groups.

Joanne is a 50-year-old part-time office worker. She is separated from her husband, and her grown up children no longer live at home. Her widowed mother, May, now lives with her having found it difficult to cope in her own home due to her failing memory. May now requires a great deal of caring for, and, although Joanne is managing with the help of neighbours, she does find it a great strain. Her mother goes into the local hospital occasionally to give her a break, and, although May does not like being in hospital, understandably, the break is very important for Joanne. Joanne will tell her own story.

'Although I needed the break from Mum, I did feel very guilty at first when she went into hospital. I really felt I needed to talk to someone about what I felt about Mum – even though I wasn't sure what I was feeling half the time – a mixture of love, pity, affection, frustration and I must admit fury and rage sometimes. I talked to the nurses and a social worker at different times, but though they were sometimes kind, they always gave me advice or encouragement which looking back I realise I didn't want. Anyway, once when I was visiting Mum during one of her 'breaks' in hospital, I met Dorothy, whose Dad was also on the ward for holiday relief. We got chatting and ended up going for a coffee. We just chatted about our experiences, but I can't tell you what a relief it was to talk to someone who really **understood** what it was like. I could tell her how furious and hateful I sometimes felt towards Mum, without worrying about what she might think about me, because I know she felt the same things. It seems so simple now, but before then I just felt so confused and guilty about what I was feeling. Once it was out in the open it didn't seem so bad. We also talked about the good things, but it was being able to show feelings which I was just frightened to show to others that made all the difference. I still see Dorothy regularly, although her father has since died. I think she found it helpful to talk to me when that happened as well. Altogether we've been a great help to each other.'

Joanne's story shows a few things. Firstly a carer is likely to experience a number of powerful and sometimes contradictory feelings at the same time. Love and anger, pity and affection, for example. And these feelings may be hard to express to other people, especially the negative feelings like anger: 'What will people think of me if I tell them I hate my father sometimes when he's being difficult?'

Another painful feeling experienced by many carers involves **grief.** It can be that an elderly confused relative has changed so much that the carer feels the the 'real' person has died, and so the carer starts grieving for the loss of the relative, even while still caring for him or her.

Finding someone who will **understand** and, more importantly, **accept** what you feel can therefore be very important for a carer. Making contact with other people should not be difficult. Voluntary organisations like the Alzheimer's Disease Society, Age Concern, and Help the Aged may well have relative support groups, and this is sometimes true also of social services and hospitals. It's often only by phoning around and asking, or by contacting the Citizens' Advice Bureau, that people find out.

Whatever the person does, the idea is not that this kind of pain can be removed, but rather that it can be brought out in the open, understood and accepted, rather than bottled up.

Difficulties with mood. Relating to the 'pain' discussed above, many also experience other sorts of emotional problems, depression and anxiety being the main ones: we'll look at each in turn.

Depression. The main sign of depression is of course feeling sad and 'low'. Other less obvious ones include difficulty sleeping, loss of appetite, reduction in drive or 'get up and go', and preoccupation with worries. There are likely to be a number of possible causes including the pain and grief discussed above. Another important cause will be that carers often have to reduce their activities – hobbies and interests – in order to look after a relative. As these activities are often crucial in terms of our general level of enjoyment of life, to reduce them or cut them out altogether will inevitably lead to a person's mood being affected. Some carers realise this and have to be very firm about maintaining their interests.

George looks after his wife, Glynis, who is very confused and needs a great deal of assistance and attention.

'When Glynis first became ill, I spent most of my time looking after her. I had been a keen bowls player, but it seemed callous to carry on when Glynis was so unwell. Of course it turned out that Glynis wasn't really going to get better, that I was going to be looking after her for quite some time. The upshot was that I didn't get back to playing bowls. The problem was that I was really very keen on playing – since retirement it was the most important thing outside of home. And of course it was great to be with the other blokes. When I was looking after Glynis I missed it a lot, and I felt resentful towards her, though God knows it wasn't her fault was it?! I thought in the end blow it! You've got to have some pleasure, especially when the rest of your life is so difficult, so I arranged with Age Concern that a volunteer would come and sit with Glynis once or twice a week, so I can go off and have a game. Glynis didn't like it – she gets a bit nervous when I'm out – but I've put my foot down and stuck to it, and she's not so bad now. And it certainly gives me a fair bit of pleasure like before – it's really something to look forward to every week.'

George's story shows how easy it is to slip out of the habit of just 'doing things' which are often taken for granted, but which are very important for our self-esteem. Once we get out of the habit of doing things, it may take a big effort to get going again. But it is possible, and it is important to keep our spirits high, especially, as George points out, when other parts of life are difficult. We need to balance out the negative experiences with positive ones. The difficulty is that the negative ones come easily, whereas the positive ones often have to be worked at. The important principle at work here is that our mood generally changes as a result of what we do (or don't do). This is the opposite of what people usually believe: 'If only I felt a bit brighter I'd be able to go out and enjoy myself'. Although that statement seems to make sense, it does seem that the reverse is closer to reality. In other words we'd do better to say 'I feel awful so I'll go out and enjoy myself and then I'll feel better.' We can all remember times when we've not wanted to go out, but we've forced ourselves (or been forced), and ended up enjoying ourselves. It's the same principle – behaviour changes mood. The implication of this for carers is that they have to be particularly careful to ensure that they maintain at least one regularly enjoyable activity, even though this may seem selfish, (it isn't of course) and even though it may be difficult to arrange. It is vital that the needs of the carer are met as well as that of the person being cared for.

Anxiety. Feelings of nervousness and emotional tension are very common in carers. In the next section we'll look at how the emotional or psychological feelings of nervousness are tied in to a person's level of physical tension.

The physical strain

If we find ourselves in any situation in which we have to work hard without much of a break, and where the work has only low levels of satisfaction involved, then we are likely to become more tense **physically.** This sounds obvious, but what in fact is going on in the body is very complex. Hormones (such as adrenalin) are released into the blood stream to increase bodily activity, such that muscle tension increases, blood pressure increases, respiration rate increases, heart rate increases. These changes can happen at levels where the person does not recognise it. If we are facing stresses like an interview, or examination, or driving test, then we'll almost certainly notice the high levels, but when the stress is less extreme, but more long-term, then the bodily changes are still happening, but are not noticed. This is likely to be the case with carers, who are often experiencing continual stress day in and day out. The effects of this on the body will be quite powerful but probably not very specific. The continual increase in muscle tension will probably show itself through physical tiredness, aches and pains, and tension headaches in particular. Increased heart rate will make people feel 'nervy' and anxious. The effects of the various hormones and other chemicals that are released into the bloodstream will be to make the person feel generally tense, irritable, and not able to 'switch off' and relax, even when they have a chance to relax. Obviously we all feel stressed and have the above experiences from time to time. The problem is that for some carers this is happening to them virtually **all** the time.

Coping with physical strain. The physical reactions to stress outlined above seem very negative, but the existence of such a stress response is to help us cope with difficulties and danger by alerting our bodies to help us overcome them. This is also called the 'fight or flight' response. Human beings have evolved with this because throughout history we have lived in very dangerous environments. The need to respond to danger in the form of predators, or other humans, was therefore developed and passed on. In these less dangerous times we no longer need such a well-developed stress response, but it will be a long time before our physical evolution catches up with our social environment. In the meantime we are prone to responding very physically to stress. So what can we do to counter these reactions, especially for those of us (like carers) who are experiencing continuous tension?

One obvious answer is to relax, and in fact this simple-sounding activity can be very useful if it is taken seriously, so we'll be looking at relaxation later.

Exercise. However, before relaxation, there is another approach that is likely to be useful. The clue to this lies in the fact that the stress response is, in effect, preparing us for activity – 'fight or flight'. As we've seen we don't need to fight or flee in situations nowadays, but our bodies are basically prepared for us to do so. If we don't, we carry on in this state of preparation with the various ill-effects (such as tiredness) noted above. The solution is to arrange to use the energy which your body has created and which needs expression. In other words, exercise! Exercise will help to 'burn off' the various effects of the stress response, and so allow the body to return to a state of relative relaxation. The best exercises are those that involve all or most of the muscles of the body, but which also increase the activity of the heart and lungs, in other words they make you become breathless – a sign that you are using your heart and lungs, not just your muscles. Exercises that combine these functions – using muscles **and** heart/lungs – include swimming, jogging, aerobics and general keep-fit programmes. Swimming is one of the best, as it is excellent for developing the efficiency of the heart and lungs, and though it exercises a number of muscles, it does not strain them (which is possible with the other exercises if insufficient care is taken).

Of course for people starting to exercise for the first time, especially older people, great care must be taken to start very gradually, preferably under the guidance of a qualified instructor, and after a check-up with your G.P. If these precautions are taken, the benefits can be very considerable.

The following account comes from Pam, whose story we read at the beginning of this chapter.

'A friend of mine had discussed exercising, as she'd started going to keep-fit classes at a local community centre. She'd always been a bit nervy, but she seemed so much calmer that I thought I'd have a go, especially as I'd been feeling so tense and irritable looking after John. Unfortunately I couldn't do keep-fit, as I've quite bad arthritis in both knees. Luckily I noticed that the local swimming pool were advertising special sessions giving adults swimming lessons, so I plucked up courage and went along. I was very self-conscious at first as I'm a bit overweight, but after a while that didn't seem to matter and I started to enjoy it after the first few lessons. I also felt the benefit when I got home – I really felt a lot better, calmer and better able to cope. Despite that, it's still a real effort to get to the pool, as I never feel like going, (it's quite a long bus ride) so I really have to push myself. Once I'm there it's fine, and I'm certainly getting the benefit now.'

Relaxation. As we mentioned above, relaxation is a misleadingly simple word. To become deeply relaxed is probably a state that few people manage to achieve today. Many of us feel we are relaxed when we're slumped in front of the television, but if our level of muscular tension was measured, it would probably show that we are far from truly relaxed. In other words proper relaxation is a state that requires some effort and practice, and isn't necessarily something that comes naturally, especially if we are already tense, and even more so if we have been tense for some time. The effects of deep relaxation are very significant: heart rate and blood pressure are reduced, muscles are freed of much tension, breathing is gentle and regular, stress-related chemicals are absent from the bloodstream, the person feels calm and relaxed.

Learning deep relaxation. The first thing is to see relaxation as a **skill**. That is, it involves learning a technique that will take time and practice before the person feels significant benefit.

The appendix at the end of this book contains instructions for a straightforward set of relaxation exercises known as progressive deep muscle relaxation exercises. The exercises go through each muscle group in turn with the person alternatively tensing and then relaxing the muscle in question. This has been found to be a very effective way of reducing tension in muscles, and, once each muscle group is relaxed in this way, the whole body is affected in the way outlined above: reduced heart rate and so on. In other words **muscular** relaxation is the key to general deep relaxation.

Exercise is important in combination with relaxation for the following reasons. Firstly the stress chemicals released into the bloodstream need to be burned off by exercise, as they tend to stay in the bloodstream otherwise. Relaxation is therefore easier after exercise. Secondly the muscle groups will be 'naturally' tired after exercise (unlike the drained feeling after feeling tense all day), again making relaxation easier. Finally the sense of well-being that people experience after exercise is important and useful in preparing for relaxation.

Starting a relaxation and exercise programme. Having first checked with your G.P., decide which exercise is most practical and most interesting for you. Choose one which won't involve too much trouble to organise, and which will fit in with your own work schedule. If exercising for the first time, try and arrange for lessons in whatever form of exercise you have chosen. Whatever the exercise, the principle should be to start with very little, and to build up gradually.

As for relaxation, the exercises at the end of this book can be used. Initially they may be hard to follow, especially as you will be trying to read them at the same time. However, after some practice, you should be able to memorise them. Alternatively, there are a number of commercial relaxation tapes available in many shops, particularly health food shops, and this is often an easier way to learn relaxation. Whatever method you use, it is important to make relaxation easier by doing it when you feel less tense – after exercise as mentioned above, or after a hot bath, or when you have some time to yourself. All this is difficult if you have a relative to care for, but building an exercise/relaxation programme into your life is possible, even though it may take careful organisation and planning. The benefits for a carer are likely to be great.

To conclude, stress and strain in someone who is caring for a relative is likely to be considerable. The combination of different emotional strains and physical stress may seem overpowering. However we hope this chapter has shown that, by looking at the different sorts of stress and strain individually rather than experiencing them as an overwhelming whole, the carer can tackle at least some of them. The greater the stress the carer is experiencing, the more difficult it is to put into action a programme to deal with it. But it is when stress is stronger that it is most important. The best thing is to tackle stresses gradually and one at a time, concentrating on the things that **can** be done. However nearly all carers need a lot of external help. This is usually provided by friends, relatives or neighbours. If this support is not possible, people then have to rely on the health and social services, so in the next chapter we will look at this area in more detail.

8 Services for elderly people and their carers

For a carer with a confused relative or friend, understanding all the various services that there are must seem virtually impossible as it is so complex. So this chapter is intended as a rough guide to the services available.

Before discussing the provision of services, it is important to remember the points raised in Chapter 1, in which we discussed the power of ageism in today's society. Unfortunately, Health and Social Service professionals and the private and voluntary sector are in no way immune from this in terms of their attitudes to elderly people and their carers. This means that it is difficult to predict the kind of response elderly people and their carers are likely to receive from different individuals in the system. For example, one G.P. may respond to a carer's request for assistance with an elderly confused relative by saying 'it's just old age' or 'there's nothing I can do', and may rely on referral to a social worker to arrange admission to an old people's home. Another G.P. may respond with genuine concern, and will help organise a variety of services to maintain the elderly person at home. It is therefore likely that a mixture of attitudes will be found in all services for elderly people, so an additional burden on a carer is to try and ensure that the professional(s) with whom he or she is dealing are not content with providing a second or third rate service to elderly people. This can mean having to be particularly assertive with some professionals in order to badger people into providing effective treatment, so this area will be looked at in more detail at the end of this chapter.

There are three basic 'strands' of provision, so we will provide a description of the services that each strand provides. The three strands are 1) the Health Service, 2) the Social Services, and 3) the private and voluntary sector.

Health Service provision for elderly people and their carers

The primary care team. For most people, the first point of contact with services is their G.P. The G.P. can be seen as the gatekeeper to a number of community-based health professionals, usually known as the primary care team. We will list those services which are often part of primary care teams:

a) **The district nurse**: Provides nursing care at home, such as doing dressings, giving advice to carers about lifting, helping with bathing and washing. The district nurse will also check on the general physical health of the person.

b) **The health visitor**: Provides advice about health matters at home, such as diet, constipation, incontinence.

c) **Incontinence adviser**: Most district authorities now have a specially trained nurse contactable through your G.P. who provides specific help with incontinence problems. The incontinence adviser will be able to advise on various incontinence aids such as waterproof underclothes, disposable, absorbent pads and plastic sheets to cover mattresses, which are available to minimise discomfort and reduce laundry costs. She will also be able to help on other aspects of dealing with incontinence and liaise with the district nursing service. A laundry service to carers may be available in your area.

d) **The community psychiatric nurse**: Provides nursing care for elderly people who are experiencing psychological problems.

e) **The chiropodist**: Provides foot care.

f) **The clinical psychologist**: Provides services to people (including elderly) with psychological problems, employing a variety of therapeutic approaches, and often involving the family in treatment. (Clinical Psychology is the smallest profession in the N.H.S., so many areas have few psychologists involved in services for elderly people.)

Social workers are also likely to relate closely to the primary care team, which may also be able to call on the services of other professions, such as speech therapists, physiotherapists and occupational therapists, though these tend to be more hospital-based.

The acute hospital. If you are a carer requiring help looking after an elderly relative, your doctor may ask one or more of the above professionals to provide assistance. However, if the problem is such that more specific (usually medical) help is needed, then the person may be referred to the hospital services. For elderly people, the most significant medical personnel will be the following:

a) **The geriatrician**: A doctor who has specialised in the physical ailments of old age.

b **The neurologist**: A doctor who specialises in physical disorders of the brain and nervous system.

c) **The psychiatrist**: A doctor who specialises in mental illness in any age group.

d) **The psychogeriatrician**: A doctor who specialises in mental illness in elderly people.

e **Others**: Include doctors who specialise in a variety of areas, such as the heart, the bones, etc, and who may be required to treat elderly people with problems in these areas.

Non-medical personnel.

a) **Physiotherapists**: Specialising in improving mobility and general physical functioning in elderly people.

b) **Occupational therapists**: Dealing with helping elderly people recover/maintain activities (e.g. cooking) following illness, as well as providing 'diversional' activities.

c) **Speech therapists**: Specialists in helping people recover language abilities, usually following strokes.

d) **Clinical psychologists**: (Already described above).

e) **Nursing staff**: Providing basic nursing care and support.

An elderly person being referred to the acute hospital service will usually see one of the medical specialists first, either as an out-patient at hospital, or, more rarely, on a home visit. If the problem can be treated at home, the person will be seen at an out-patient clinic. If more intensive help is needed, then the person may attend a day hospital for a (usually) limited period of time to receive treatment. In addition, the medical specialist is likely to involve some of the above staff, for example physiotherapy may be given at the day hospital for elderly people.

When problems are more serious, an elderly person may be admitted to a ward under the care of a particular medical specialist, depending on the nature of the problem. For example, someone with serious psychological problems may be admitted through the psychiatrist or psychogeriatrician, whereas an elderly person who has suffered a stroke is likely to be admitted to a special ward for elderly people under the care of a geriatrician. Whatever the specialist, there again will be a variety of non-medical professionals involved in looking after elderly patients, helping them to recover their level of functioning.

However, if the physical or psychological problems do not respond to these therapeutic endeavours, and if there is little chance of returning home, then elderly people may be moved on to the next part of the hospital service, the long-stay ward.

Within the acute hospital service, the potential for confusion is very high, with different doctors treating different 'parts' of a person, and sometimes with patchy communication between them, so services can vary from place to place, depending on the relationships that have been built up. The G.P. is often seen as the central figure in terms of the linking of services, but again there can be patchy communication between hospital and G.P. practices, with a lack of clarity concerning the co-ordination of an individual's treatment. Of course, the interest and commitment of a G.P. to his or her elderly patients can vary enormously. One G.P may be involved in building up a good support network of staff to help keep an elderly confused person at home, whilst another will pressurise elderly confused patients and relatives to admit the person to an old people's home.

Long-term care (see also Chapter 9). Sometimes an elderly person will be admitted to an acute ward for treatment, but even after treatment they remain very disabled. If there is no chance of going home or back to the community generally, that person may well be transferred to a long-stay or 'continuing care' ward. These are wards where medical and nursing input is concerned with keeping patients as well as possible physically, although often there is very little in the way of activities or any kind of additional therapy, such as speech therapy and physiotherapy. The consultant in charge of the wards may be either a geriatrician or a psychiatrist/psychogeriatrician, although medical staff often have little day-to-day involvement in these wards, since the patients there have not responded to medical input.

Some districts will have developed more community based services for elderly people, although these are the exception and not the rule so far. These services may take the form of community teams, where a variety of disciplines come together regularly in order to pool resources to try and enable elderly people in need to stay at home. The community team should be based in or near the primary care setting, so that it is close to the people who will use the service. However, as we mentioned above, so far this sort of team is relatively unusual, and we will look at the reasons for this later in the chapter. We will now go on to look at the Social Service strand of provision for elderly people.

The Social Services

We can split the provision provided by the Social Services into two areas: 1) the personal social services and 2) residential and day care services. We will review each in turn.

Personal Social Services. These are the services provided for people usually in their own home. For elderly people, this will primarily involve home helps, meal-on-wheels and arranging the payment of benefits. An elderly person or carer requiring social service support can apply to their local Social Service office (or alternatively a G.P. or other health professional may refer them) after which a social worker will visit to assess the need for services. Social workers are 'gatekeepers' to this part of the system in a way similar to G.P.s in the primary care and hospital system.

a) **Home help service**: Provides help with things like getting up, dressing, preparing meals, shopping and general housework. Increasingly home help services are available in the evenings and at weekends. Some even provide a night sitting service.

b) **Aids and adaptation service**: Provides aids for daily living or adaptations to the home aimed at helping a disabled person achieve maximum independence. Walking frames, wheelchairs, chemical toilets/commodes should be available as well as bathroom aids (seats, boards, mats, nails), dressing aids (velcro fastenings, and aids to help putting on clothes) and feeding aids (special cutlery, plates, cups, bowls). For adaptations of the home, grants may be available. An occupational therapist should help in making an assessment of your needs.

c) **Welfare Rights Service**: Provides information and assistance on a whole range of benefits, entitlements and services. The Welfare Rights Officer can check that your means tested benefits, income support and caring benefit are correct and can even offer help with fuel problems, negotiating with gas and electricity boards on your behalf and even represent for you at Social Security and Medical Appeals Tribunals.

The main benefits available to people with dementia and their carers are the following:

(i) **Attendance Allowance**: This is a benefit paid to a person who needs a lot of help and supervision because of mental or physical disability. It is paid on two rates depending on whether the disabled person needs looking after day **and** night (higher rate) or during the day **or** night (lower rate). The rules state that the disabled person, in order to qualify, must require help with basic bodily functions (for example, eating, drinking, toileting, walking, washing and so on) or would be in substantial danger without the attendance of someone else. Attendance allowance is tax-free but is not paid to those people in state funded or aided residential care like hospitals, old people's homes or private homes where an elderly person is receiving income support to pay towards the cost of that care.

(ii) **Invalid Care Allowance**: This is a weekly cash allowance paid to the carer who has to stay at home to look after someone who qualifies for attendance allowance. Both men **and** women are eligible, **married** or single, but you must be under pensionable age (65 for a man, 60 for a woman) **before** you start to claim (this makes over 40 per cent of all carers ineligible – again mostly women who happen to be of pensionable age). You must spend at least 35 hours a week caring for the disabled person but you do not necessarily have to be a relative or even to live at the same address. Invalid Care Allowance is not affected by the amount of your savings (i.e. it is not means tested) but it does count as taxable income. Currently, you must not be doing work for which you earn more than £20 a week after deductions in order to qualify.

(iii) **Mobility Allowance**: This is another non-means tested cash benefit aimed at helping severely disabled people to become more mobile. It is paid to the disabled person who must **not** have reached their sixty-sixth birthday before applying. This benefit is payable up to the age of seventy-five, as long as the person is incapable of walking and likely to remain so for at least a year.

(iv) **Invalidity Benefit**: This paid to people who because of illness are still unable to work after their sickness benefit comes to an end. However, it only payable to people who become disabled **before** reaching the age of sixty for men and fifty-five for women.

There are a whole number of other social security and housing benefits, tax allowances and other entitlements. For further information contact your Welfare Rights Officer through your local Social Services office. Alternatively the Citizen's Advice

Bureaux or organisations like Age Concern should be able to help. Their addresses are available in the Appendix.

Residential and day care services. Social Service departments often run and organise day care facilities for elderly people, ranging from informal luncheon clubs, to fully staffed day centres catering for a large number of people. These day centres usually function as social centres, although they may have additional therapist input from Health and Social Service staff (occupational therapists, for example). Referral to day facilities is obtained through the social worker.

The social services own and run a large number of old people's homes (also called Part III accommodation following the 1948 National Assistance Act). These homes vary in size and number, with the average numbers of places per authority falling between thirty and sixty.

Social Service homes are sometimes used to provide relative relief (also called respite care). This is when elderly people enter an old people's home for a short stay to give the carer a break (this service is also offered by some hospitals).

There are fewer homes being built these days by local (Social Services) authorities, partly due to the cost and partly because these homes have been increasingly seen as not providing an acceptably high quality of life. However, there has been a mushrooming recently of private (that is profit-making) residential homes which have to be registered with local authorities, whose job it is to ensure minimal standards in these establishments. We will look at this third strand next.

The private and voluntary sector

The mushrooming of the private sector has taken place over the past few years primarily because of changes in the way benefits are paid. Without going into detail, what this means is that the owner of a private (registered) home can or will be paid about £160 per week (at the time of writing) to look after an elderly person, assuming that person does not possess assets above a certain level.

Private homes do vary a great deal in terms of the quality of life they provide, and the enormous increase in their numbers has put an additional demand on the local authorities, whose job it is to check that homes have minimum standards before allowing registration. Private homes do tend to be smaller than local authority homes, which can be important in terms of how pleasant they are to live in. However, they are of course run strictly for profit, and so many are unwilling to take more disabled elderly people (except for more specialist and expensive nursing homes) and few are likely to employ additional staff (for example for occupational therapy, physiotherapy, or speech therapy) to improve the residents' levels of functioning and activities.

There are also other homes which are not profit-making, being run by charitable organisations, often for specific groups of retired people, such as actors, or people of certain religious denominations. This brings us to the increasing importance of the voluntary sector.

Voluntary organisations and services. In some ways the word 'voluntary' is misleading, as increasingly some of the charities are relatively powerful and well financed, employing significant numbers of people to help run the organisations, recruit and train volunteers, produce planning documents, and so on. Probably the largest and best known are MIND (not specifically for the elderly), Age Concern and Help the Aged.

Current trends have resulted in voluntary groups being far more involved in planning and providing services alongside the Health and Social Services than was hitherto the case. These services include day centres, 'sitting' and visiting services, and in some areas managing residential services as well. Many areas also have relative support groups which are run by voluntary agencies.

Since the organisations are predominantly voluntary, they do vary significantly from place to place in terms of the level of provision. This means that a carer needs to find out what is happening in his or her own area, and probably the best way to do this is via the local Citizens' Advice Bureau, or Social Services department.

E

Some problems with health, social, private and voluntary services

One major criticism of services for elderly people is that they tend to segregate elderly people from the rest of society. Facilities such as old people's homes, geriatric wards, elderly day centres, are often the foundation of statutory services, and yet they segregate elderly people, often making difficult or preventing (albeit unintentionally) contact with other younger people including friends and family. If we think about it carefully, the very last thing that an elderly confused person needs is to be surrounded by people who are also elderly and confused. It is vitally important that someone who is confused has social contact, and social contact with a person who can help focus the confused person's talk, and reinforce them when they talk clearly. By placing elderly confused people together, we ensure that their social environment is confusing. Often we find non-confused and confused elderly people in the same setting, especially in old people's homes. We could say that, in this case, the non-confused will be able to help the confused. In fact, what usually happens is that elderly alert people do not want to be reminded of what condition might await them. They do not want to see the negative consequences of old age any more than is necessary, so they will often tend to avoid confused people in homes, wards, day centres and day hospitals.

Unfortunately, the trend is for services to become increasingly specialised, the psychogeriatric service being a recent medical specialism. The services will tend to segregate people, particularly as they tend to be what is called 'buildings led'; that is, once finance for a new service has been agreed, the first step by planners is usually to erect a building, the second step to fill it with staff, then thirdly put the patients in the building and hope that somehow things will turn out all right. Obviously, this is something of a caricature, but is essentially true of most services. Services which are more sensitive to the needs of elderly people are being started in different parts of the country, and these services usually aim at helping keep people in their own homes, often despite serious multiple handicaps. Some schemes provide residential accommodation in ordinary housing, rather than large institutions, with nursing or other staff living in and providing the necessary support.

These schemes are few and far between so far, but there is currently a greater emphasis on community care, and also on consumer/carer involvement, and both these factors could help generate new and better services, although the piecemeal approach of successive governments to community care is a serious hindrance in this.

How the carer can use services

For the carer and elderly relative at present, the above points may not be of great immediate relevance. For them it is important to find out what is available now to assist them in their current situation.

Perhaps the first thing to do is to identify what help you need. If you have an elderly relative who seems to be becoming confused, then clearly the first thing to do is to get a thorough medical examination. This can be done by the G.P., or he or she may refer you to a specialist, usually a geriatrician. Some G.P.s may not seem to be particularly concerned because, as we have already suggested, negative attitudes to old age are often found in Health and Social Service staff as well. If this is the case, then possible solutions are simply to be assertive and persistent with your G.P., or alternatively change to one who will be more sympathetic.

In any case, a medical examination is essential. Once this is done, you should be told of what the cause of the confusion is, and any reversible conditions (such as we discussed in Chapter 4) will be treated. However, if the elderly person's confusion is due to brain damage of a kind that is irreversible, then the carer will need to discover what help is available. One problem likely to be encountered is that, at present, many of our services tend to be crisis-related. That is, Health and Social Services often avoid becoming involved with helping a carer until that carer has 'had enough'. By that time, things may have reached such a pitch that little can be done to keep the elderly person at home, as the carer is at the end of his or her tether, and so the elderly person is admitted to hospital or a 'home'. To try and overcome this, carers often have to be very assertive to obtain the help they need.

It is important to work out what help the carer needs to keep going without suffering more stress than is necessary. We've looked at ways of coping in Chapter 7, but it's also important to find out which services can help as well.

Local voluntary groups such as Age Concern will help you to identify what voluntary services are available, which may help reduce the amount of stress faced. Many carers find a simple sitting service is priceless in terms of giving one or two free periods each week, helping them to look after their own needs. Some carers may need additional help, for example having a longer break from looking after their relatives. The relative may need to go into residential care, such as a hospital ward or old people's home, as many areas offer 'holiday relief' for carers for one or two week periods.

Health and Social Services often have day centres/hospitals which can care for elderly people up to five days a week. A carer who feels this may be a solution would need to contact a social worker via the local Social Services department (for Social Service day centre) or again contact the G.P. for a referral to day hospitals.

Although we have looked at several of the difficulties in going into wards, homes and day centres, the fact is that many carers desperately need these breaks, so, as often the only way this need can be met is to be admitted to a residential service or day centre, this has got to be accepted. A distraught carer is neither helping themselves nor their relative.

As we indicated above, it does take quite a lot of effort to find one's way around the services, and often the best help is to find someone in a similar position who has experience of the process. The voluntary services can be very useful in bringing people together in this way.

9 Residential care

Introduction

Throughout this book we have stressed the importance of maintaining the place in the community of an elderly person with dementia. We have also at times been critical of the past history and current record of residential care for the elderly. This is because we feel there are special problems with this kind of provision, although we do of course recognise the dedication and expertise of many of the individual staff who operate and work in the residential homes and this is particularly the case in the private sector.

There will always be the need for some forms of residential care, even with well-developed community services, as some people simply cannot be maintained in their own home and others may consciously choose to enter residential care of their own free will. We should say, however, that our own experience tells us that the number of elderly people, with or without dementia, who freely choose to enter residential care is small. The more usual case is for relatives and family to find themselves seeking care because of the deteriorated condition of the elderly person, or an elderly person seeking care because they feel they have become a burden on others.

The decision to move

Giving up one's own home and moving permanently to a residential home is an extremely important step and one that has to be very carefully thought through by an elderly person and his or her family. This is particularly the case for confused people whose remaining links to reality may consist of the familiar objects, spaces and atmosphere of a house where they have lived for many years. There is a good deal of evidence to suggest that elderly people find the stress of relocation to a hospital or residential home difficult to bear and that this is magnified if the old person is under coercion to leave, or at least not fully involved in the decision to move and the transition process itself.

Despite what was said earlier in Chapter 1 about the bulk of resources provided for elderly people going into residential care, the reality for a family seeking a residential placement for a seriously disabled older relative is that such a place is often very difficult to obtain. Such a family may find, for example, that local authority old people's homes in their area are heavily over-subscribed and that a formal or informal waiting list is in operation. Social workers may be reluctant to advise relatives on options for private care for legal and ideological reasons, leaving relatives with little information on what to do next. Admission to a hospital bed will depend on a consultant's opinion on whether treatment is needed or possible, or whether an old person's problems are severe enough to require the allocation of a scarce long-term hospital bed. Few hospitals have a significant number of long-term beds and many of the older hospitals where such facilities were located are now in the process of being 'run down' and closed as part of the government's policy on community care.

Perhaps the most difficult and important point about the decision to opt for residential care is to be honest, with yourself and the elderly person, as to who the move is for. Many of the alleged benefits of residential care for the elderly are more mythical than real. One reason often given by families for seeking a residential place is to alleviate the loneliness and isolation felt by an elderly relative who lives alone. However, it is well known that residential establishments can be extremely lonely places. Generally, studies on old peoples' homes find that social contact and companionship are not necessarily increased by moving to residential care. Anyone who has spent a considerable time living in a hotel, for example, can testify to the sense of loneliness that can be experienced as a result of living with strangers.

Another apparent advantage of residential care is that in such establishments there will always be someone to 'look after' an elderly person around the clock. Unfortunately such assumptions may be misplaced in residential homes where, because of the number of residents and shortages of staff, supervision may be perfunctory. Accidents can and do happen in residential homes as they do elsewhere. In fact the evidence suggests that an elderly person is more likely to have an accident, such as a fall, in residential environments than they are in their own homes. Staff in residential homes will generally operate in such a way as to minimise accidents occurring. However, if not enough staff are available for proper supervision, then other strategies will be used to keep residents 'safe'. These vary from the imposition of rules, regulations and restrictions to excessive sedation and tranquillisation of residents. There is therefore a potential cost to be paid for a safe environment and this cost is often borne by the old person for the sake of relatives' peace of mind.

Taking an elderly person into your own home

It is quite natural that relatives should seek to protect the old person from the worst effects of their illness. Caring for a dementing elderly person in their own home is a difficult business especially when, as so often happens, the main responsibilities fall on one carer. Habitual ways of responding to problems develop which may militate against the long-term ability of that carer to cope. For example, in response to pressing demands arising from the old person's behaviour, a carer may find herself visiting many times a day, locking the old person in or taking on the role of punchbag for aggressive and angry neighbours.

In such circumstances a family may well consider having the old person come to live with them or even selling the carer's and the old person's house with a view to buying a large house to accommodate the extended family. This may be felt to be preferable to putting an old person into residential care. However, it is not very realistic to expect a person with dementia to stick to his or her own part of the house or to imagine that things will necessarily be easier because the old person is under the same roof. Of course carers may not have the encumbrance of frequent visits, but neither will they be able to 'get away' from problems. Typically, arrangements where a demented old person comes to live with carers result in an **increased** dependence of the old person on their support and **increased** conflict as the old person's rhythms and routines run into conflict with the needs of others in the household. The needs of other family members, especially children and teenagers, should be very carefully considered. Finally, it should be remembered that, whatever community statutory support is available by way of home helps, social workers and nursing services, it is likely to be scarce and will tend to be directed towards those who live alone rather than those who have family living with them.

The main types of residential care

Local Authority old People's Homes (also called 'Part III' homes because they are described under Part III of the National Assistance Act (1948). We have already discussed some of the original aims of these establishments and some of the problems with the care they offer. The homes aim to meet the needs of frail but mentally alert old people although in the past twenty years the average resident in such homes has become much more disabled. It is increasingly those whose disabilities can no longer be coped with in a community setting who become candidates for local authority residential care. It is estimated that over a half of residents in old people's homes are 'confused' or suffering from dementia, yet few staff have any specialist skills or training in these conditions. Inadequate resources, poor staffing levels, in combination with increased levels of dependency in many homes, make it impossible for staff to provide a good service, despite good intentions. No guidelines exist on what proportion of 'confused' people can be accommodated in such a home whilst still providing a reasonable standard of care.

Many homes have improved the quality of the physical and social environment, for example, by the provision of more single room accommodation, a more sensitive appreciation of the importance of possessions, greater choice at mealtimes and the reorganisation of the building into smaller 'group living' units. Such enlightened arrangements vary from one authority to another and even between homes under the same authority.

In some parts of the country so-called 'specialist' homes for the mentally infirm or confused may exist. A particular part or 'wing' of an ordinary residential home may be sectioned off for the same purpose. The idea behind these segregated units is usually to provide higher levels of staffing and resources and to do this most efficiently by gathering the most confused or mentally disordered people together. However, doubts about the concept of specialist or segregated homes have increased. Maintaining a reasonably ordered environment and retaining staff can be a problem with highly mentally disabled residents. Another danger is that 'specialist' homes may become 'dumping grounds' for difficult and troublesome residents as well as those suffering from dementia.

Many local authorities use old people's homes to offer 'short stay' or 'holiday relief' admissions for elderly people being supported by their family in the community. 'Rotating care' is an arrangement where an old person is admitted to an old people's home at regular intervals for a short stay and then returned to the community. These relatively new schemes can be very useful to the carers of elderly people with dementia, although the effect, of course, is to reduce further the number of beds available for long-term placement.

An application for admission to an old people's home can only be made by a social worker. Decisions about suitability for admission will be taken by a group of social services officers, sometimes with advice from other health professionals. If the need is urgent, arrangements for admission will be made immediately. More usually an old person may have to wait a considerable period for a place. Much depends on when and where a bed becomes available. Immediate admission may be to a home in a part of the authority distant from family and friends. On the other hand, sticking to a request for a genuinely local placement might require a wait of weeks or months.

Social workers should be able to give guidance on whether an application would be likely to be successful. Admission policies do differ from area to area. Some authorities will not consider elderly people with significant confusion, incontinence or physical handicaps that might require intensive staffing. Quite reasonably, social services have to consider the effect on other residents and on the organisation of the home of admitting other highly dependent people, when the home may be unreasonably overburdened with disability and understaffed.

Care in an old people's home is not free and this can come as quite a shock to relatives. Costs are decided on the basis of a means test of the old person's assets and a detailed financial assessment is usually required. Decisions on charges payable are complex and to some extent at the discretion of individual authorities. However, an old person will be asked to pay costs on the basis of what the local authority thinks he or she can afford which, if the person has personal savings of any significance or property assets, may be up to the full cost of board, lodgings and care. Details of charges are given in the DHS booklet *Residential homes: charging and assessment* which is available from social security or social services offices.

This means that an old person may be required to sell their home to release assets to pay for the care. It is therefore important to check carefully what claim the local authority may have on an old person's estate and to receive advice on the financial aspects of the move to residential care. Independent advice can be obtained from organisations like the Citizens' Advice Bureaux or Age Concern. The finance officer of the local authority will also be helpful. Remember that, even if an old person has no personal savings or property assets, a large part of their State or other pensions will be taken by the local authority towards the cost of their keep. They will be left with a small 'pocket money' allowance each week for personal spending. At the time of writing this is set at about £8.

Private residential care in nursing or rest homes
Rest homes. Private residential care is by far the fastest growing sector of personal care for the elderly and its growth has been actively encouraged by government financial incentives, which provide funds to meet a certain amount of the weekly cost of care as long as the old person does not have significant assets himself.

Many private homes provide high quality care in pleasant surroundings, but the poorest care, unfortunately, is also to be found in the private sector. Under the Registered Homes Act (1983), any person wishing to operate a private residential home 'for the sole purpose of accommodating four or more elderly people' is required by law to register the home with the social services department of the local authority. This means that certain 'minimum standards' are laid down by the local authority which a private home must meet in terms of safety, fire precautions, administration, physical space and conditions. The homes must also lay themselves open to regular inspection by the registrations officer employed by the social services for this purpose. The registrations officer should have a list of all the private homes that have been registered with the authority. This list should be available on request or through your social worker.

It is firmly the responsibility of the old person and their family to decide and investigate which private home is most suitable. Neither social workers nor registration officers are at liberty to express preferences or guidance about particular establishments. It should also be noted that homes of less than four people do not have to register at all. By and large these establishments should be avoided. The fact that a home is registered is by itself no guarantee of good quality care. This is because inspections may be irregular and substandard homes may not be closed for the simple reason that there is nowhere else to accommodate the elderly people who live in them.

Use your own eyes and ears, proceed carefully, ask questions, be choosy and do not be pushed into premature decisions, even if a home, at first glance, seems to meet all your requirements. Moving into residential care is a monumental decision which, even with favourable conditions, requires difficult adjustments on the part of the old person: without such conditions a move can be disastrous. You may be surprised by the large number of private homes that are available in your area and this is to your advantage in giving more choice. However, you may find that not so many homes are willing to consider admitting a confused elderly person.

Nursing homes. Nursing homes differ from rest homes in that they undertake to provide at least one trained nurse on a twenty-four-hour basis and are registered with the health authority and inspected by them. As with rest homes there is a tremendous variation in the quality offered and there is no guarantee whatsoever that the care offered will be superior to that offered in rest homes, even though the costs of nursing homes are usually higher.

Often elderly people suffering from dementia are physically fit and not in need of 'nursing care'. Nursing homes tend to cater for clients with medical problems like immobility, severe arthritis, sickness and physical disease. The general environment may be hospital-like, perhaps with much of activity taking place in and around the residents beds rather than in the communal and social areas of the home. A nursing home may not be the most appropriate placement for a confused elderly person although this will depend on the degree of physical incapacitation shown by that person and the progression of the disease. Nursing homes may be better equipped to deal with problems like frequent incontinence, walking and co-ordination problems.

The cost of private care. The number of elderly and disabled people in residential and nursing homes who are paid for by social security payments has risen from 11,000 in 1979 to 130,000 in 1987. The total bill being paid by the government to support people in residential care was, in 1988, about £1 billion. This money is spent largely in the private sector. Private homes usually cost somewhere in the range of £150-300 a week (1988 prices) although there is considerable variation. Old people with savings of less than £3,000, and whose income is low enough to qualify for income support, have their charges at the home met up to £185 a week (at the time of writing). Those with savings of between £3,000 and £6,000 receive a reduced grant on a sliding scale. Those with savings above this figure have to pay their own way. In addition the D.H.S.S. currently gives £9.55 a week to every nursing home resident on income support.

The fact that these social security benefits are paid to claimants in private residential care without any assessment of the need for that care is an increasing target of criticism. There are fears that, as the population grows older and long-stay hospitals close, care for the elderly with dementia and others will move from large, relatively supervised institutions to small, relatively unsupervised ones, bypassing 'community care' in the process. The funding policy for residents in private homes is not likely to last indefinitely as it is becoming too expensive. The influx of cash to the private residential sector has also occurred at a time when government policy is encouraging the care of elderly people in their own homes.

Choosing a home. The most important difference between local authority and private homes is that the latter are run on a commercial basis for profit. Spending in profit-making concerns will tend towards cost effectiveness rather than quality when there is a choice to be made between them. On the other hand, state-sponsored residential care, like old people's homes, is affected by the squeeze on local authority budgets and traditional paternalistic attitudes to the care of the elderly.

Private care is not cheap so make sure you are getting value for money. Many of the aspects that make up quality of life are not easy to see at first glance and appearances can be deceptive.

You may be impressed by homes which are well presented physically, but remember that excessive cleanliness and tidiness may suggest an over-concern with things looking good. Look for a home that looks lived in rather than one that looks like a hospital, clinic or museum.

Another important aspect of quality is the calibre of staff. Try and talk to staff when visiting a home and assess their friendliness, approachability and courtesy. Do they seem to treat residents with respect and warmth? Ask the proprietor about his or her staff, how many, their backgrounds, how long do they stay. A rapid turnover of staff often reflects underlying problems in the home. Most important of all, try to spend time with residents. Ask to spend some time in a sitting area, preferably without staff being in constant attendance and talk to residents about their life in the home.

It may be useful for you to think about the following types of questions when considering the suitability of a home.

General questions. Is there reasonable access to the home by car or public transport? Are there amenities close by, such as shops, pubs, parks and so on? Is there a general sense of activity and liveliness? Are residents talking to each other? Do staff have time to talk to residents? Are there enough staff? Is the home reasonably comfortable and is there enough space to move around? Is the home designed on the basis of single bedrooms? Does it smell nice? Is there a garden? Is it used by the residents? If not, why not? In general look for a home within reasonable access that has a friendly, active atmosphere and feels comfortable, lived in and homely.

Identity. To what extent does the home reflect the fact that the old people living there are individual people with their own particular needs? Do residents have the opportunity to retain personal belongings and possessions? Do bedrooms vary in the decorations, bric-a-brac and ornaments, reflecting the fact that each has a different person living in it? Is encouragement given to people to buy items like ornaments, pictures and toiletries? Are there any practices in the home which are demeaning to an old person's self-respect, such as communal clothing or group washing and toileting? Do staff show respect for the privacy of residents? Do they knock on doors before entering, talk to the old person in a respectful way, ask permission, make sure any personal care genuinely takes place in private? In general, try to decide whether the home is sensitive to the individual needs and decisions of its residents.

Choice. Try and establish the routine of the day in the home. What choices do the residents have in what they eat, when they eat, when they get up or go to bed, when they go to the toilet or for a bath and so on? Are they asked about these things? Are their preferences acted upon? What rules and regulations apply in the home? Ask the manager directly. There is often a rule banning smoking in bedrooms, but are there any further restrictions on movement, alcohol, mixing with other residents, especially those of the opposite sex? Sometimes restrictions have to be placed on particular people for the safety of others, but do those restrictions apply to everybody regardless of their appropriateness? Are attempts made to elicit choices from residents, even confused residents? Do the staff feel this is important or of little concern? Be wary of homes which show such a lack of concern for personal choice.

Activities/independence. What activities take place in the home? Are people encouraged to maintain the skills they still have like self-care, dressing, washing, cooking, washing up and so on? Or, are the old people left to vegetate in their seats while staff cater for all their needs? Are the particular interests of residents actively encouraged, such as singing, painting, knitting or gardening? What arrangements are there to keep people mobile and exercised? What special activities are laid on for the enjoyment of residents? Finally, is there a programme, or plan, or set of goals for each individual resident and how do these plans work?

Relationships. Who do residents see from the outside world other than the staff and family visitors? How many residents go out on a regular basis? Who comes into the home from the surrounding community? What help is given to residents to get out of the home to go to the hairdresser's, shopping, seeing their doctor and so on? Can residents keep their own G.P.? Do staff make outsiders, like visitors, feel welcome? Is it possible to see a resident in privacy and are there any restrictions on visiting? In general try to ascertain the degree to which the home fosters contact and relationships between residents and staff, and between the home and the outside world.

This is a rather formidable list of questions and to some extent points to an ideal which most residential homes (private and public) will fail to meet. However, the list should serve to remind you of the necessity to go 'beyond appearances' in making an assessment of a home and to be systematic and methodical in choosing a home that you are confident will meet the old person's needs.

Long-term 'continuing care' in hospital. Hospital care of those with long-term, chronic illnesses, such as dementia, has historically been the 'Cinderella' of the National Health Service. 'Continuing care' wards usually offer a high standard of nursing and physical care but tend to be located in some of the oldest and most dilapidated hospital buildings. Many of these buildings were actually workhouses, asylums or old infirmaries, which predate the establishment of the National Health Service and tend to be very large, impersonal and daunting. Understandably, there has been pressure to demolish these buildings and establish new long-stay units of a smaller scale, close to the community of origin of the patients who live in them. However, to date, there are very few facilities of this kind in existence.

The quality of psychological and social care in hospital long-term wards is affected by the physical surroundings, negative attitudes and problems with staff recruitment and retention. In many wards, attempts are made to create a home-life atmosphere, despite the poor physical environment, by staff with positive attitudes towards elderly people and the problem of dementia. On the other hand, a luxurious facility can be manned by staff with negative attitudes. This is not to say that these staff lack care and compassion. They simply have not been shown how things could be made better.

A decision about admission to hospital will be taken by a doctor, usually a consultant psychiatrist or geriatrician. Referral to a consultant will be through the elderly person's general practitioner. The elderly person may have to attend the hospital for initial assessment. Increasingly, psychiatrists and geriatricians see people at home on this first occasion and, if the consultant feels there is a need, the old person will be taken into hospital for a further assessment. This does not mean in itself that a long-term bed will be offered. Long-term beds in hospitals have always been in great demand and because beds are scarce, an elderly person with dementia is only likely to be admitted if their problems are severe. Hospital staff may decide to seek admission to an old people's home or seek to return the old person to his or her home with some treatment and/or further support. If relatives disagree with such a decision, then it falls on them to find alternative long-term care, usually in a private home. Some hospitals will keep an old person for a time to give the relatives an opportunity to find an alternative placement.

If an elderly relative is successfully placed in a long-term hospital bed, it is very important that they continue to be seen regularly by their family. Sometimes a carer may feel that the admission is the final confirmation of their own inability to cope, and feelings of deep hurt, guilt and remorse are not uncommon. Such emotions may be accentuated by the old person's obvious unhappiness in their new environment, by the physical conditions of the ward and by the disturbed behaviour of other patients. During visits relatives may feel at a loss as to what to do and may be wary of approaching staff for fear of bothering or being a nuisance to them. The worst response to such problems is to stop visiting.

Discuss your anxieties with the staff, who will do their best to make your visits successful and who should be able to advise you on ways of helping the old person to settle and or your own emotional adjustment to the admission. Do what you can to maintain the elderly person within the family, for example, by bringing in photographs, bringing them up-to-date with news and taking grandchildren to visit. Don't be afraid to take the old person out of the ward for a walk or out of the hospital for a drive, even for a visit home, but talk to staff first about any problems that might arise. The process of adjustment to long-term care takes time both for the old person and the family, but the removal of all the stresses of caring may enable a more stable and satisfactory relationship to emerge between the elderly person and the family.

No charge is made for long-term care within National Health Service hospitals. However, an old person's state pension will be reduced after a period of time (one year) to allow a patient only a personal spending (pocket money) allowance. Other social security supplementary payments and allowances, such as attendance and invalidity benefits, will also be stopped or substantially reduced. Occupational, additional or graduated pensions are not affected. Neither are certain other pensions such as war pensions. Details of the effects on current pensions and allowances on entering long-term hospital care are contained in the booklet *Going into hospital*, available from social security offices.

The move to residential care

Finally, we will say something about the effect on an elderly person with dementia of a move from their home to a hospital or residential placement. Leaving your long-established home to enter a new, and often bewildering, environment is comparable to a bereavement or major loss in a person's life and it takes time to adjust and heal. It is sometimes claimed that, by the time an elderly person with dementia is admitted to residential care, their mental facilities have deteriorated so much that the move is of less consequence to them than to others with normal mental functioning. This claim ignores the individual differences between dementia sufferers, which we have been at pains to stress, and the varied reasons why residential care is sought. It also ignores the evidence that people with dementia 'fall back' on established and well-worn routines in a familiar environment, which are very sensitive to any subsequent change in that person's life.

There has been a good deal of study of what happens to vulnerable elderly people who move from their home into institutionalised care and this indicates that for a period following such a move they tend to show a pattern of increased sickness, passivity, depression, and decreased functioning and higher death rate compared to similarly disabled people who are not moved. However, there are important qualifications to this. Firstly, the **quality** of the environment into which they move is important in reducing the chance of these catastrophic consequences occurring. Where elderly people are moved to a **better** environment, in terms of physical comfort, warmth and support, the encouragement of independent behaviour and so on, this pattern of bad effects are not apparent. Therefore, it is important for relatives and others to determine whether the quality of the new setting will be better than the old one.

Secondly, the degree to which an old person is **prepared** and **involved** in the move is of equal importance in preventing future problems. In practice this might involve, if this is possible, the old person themselves in the decision to move. Failing this, an effort to enable the old person to understand why, how and where a move will take place should always be attempted. A more direct way of preparing an old person should be through this preparation process. Actually physically involving the old person in the move by getting them to help 'pack' their belongings , for example, can also be helpful in preparing them.

Thirdly, it is important to **minimise** as many other aspects of change as possible. Try and find a home in the same geographical locality as the person is used to. Make sure family visiting patterns are maintained as they would have been if the old person had not left their home. Maintain, as far as possible, outings, activities and any other aspects of established routine.

With these safeguards and careful planning the relocation of a confused elderly person need not lead to severe additional problems. However moving is a significant risk to an old person's well being and should be considered very carefully. It is not easy to see a respected and loved parent living in squalid conditions, perhaps causing embarrassment to some neighbours and amusement to others, to be rung by police after that parent has been found wandering in a nearby town, to have to see to the toileting and personal needs of that parent.

No criticism can be made of those who opt for residential care in these or similar conditions, although often this is the last thing a family wants. What is critical is the lack of appropriate practical, financial and emotional help or the sharing of the onerous tasks involved. However, perhaps the most courageous attitude is that which allows a person with dementia to continue to lead some resemblance of an ordinary life, with all its risks and dangers and embarrassments, in a place that is familiar and natural to them, rather than one which, through seeking to protect them, deprives them of their last remaining anchors to reality, by placing them in an institutional environment.

10 General summary

In this book we have tried to take a positive approach to the problems of dementia.

In the absence of known causes and of successful medical treatments for dementia, we have emphasised the importance of maintaining the skills and functioning of the dementia sufferer for as long as possible and the importance of maintaining such people in their familiar environments by the provision of practical community services and the support of carers.

We were particularly concerned to challenge the hopelessness that is generated by the term 'dementia' and to indicate that symptoms differ widely between sufferers and within a sufferer from time to time.

We have stressed that the terms 'dementia' and 'confusion' describe a complex of symptoms which can arise from a number of underlying diseases and medical conditions such as Alzheimer's disease and multi-infarct dementia, which are increasingly better identified but for which no cure or effective treatments exist in the majority of cases. We have described the main methods for diagnosing diseases which cause dementia and given an account of the most promising lines of research which may eventually lead to new treatments for these conditions. We have included a chapter on the major structures and functions of the brain in an attempt to help the reader understand the normal functioning of the brain and what goes wrong in the brains of people suffering from dementia. Although this material is a little technical we feel that carers, relatives and care workers should be given the opportunity to understand a disease which is usually mystifying to them.

The two main types of treatment available to dementia sufferers – drugs and behavioural approaches – are described, but it is emphasised that both work through alleviating symptoms rather than affecting the underlying disease and both have limitations. Major and minor tranquillising drugs have a very general affect on the brain, not specific to the disease, which can lead to a worsening of a sufferer's mental state and to unpleasant side-effects and dependence. Behavioural approaches call for a heavy commitment of time and energy from carers and others where no such commitment may be possible. Few health and social service workers are sufficiently skilled in the application of these techniques. However, the behavioural approach does give the reader a method for understanding the problems of individuals who suffer dementia. In general we have not given the reader rules and **advice** about how to deal with particular symptoms, simply because the expression of these symptoms will be different in each case. We therefore felt that a description of a method, with illustrations, was preferable.

Throughout the book we have tried to understand, as far as possible, something of the experience of dementia. We have tried to describe the problems of dementia, not just in terms of the effects they have on others (usually carers), but also from the viewpoint of the dementia sufferer. In this context we have at times been critical of current services, particularly of residential provision.

Finally, we have tried to view the problem of dementia within an overall picture of the response of society at large to old age and its consequences. We have drawn attention to the failure of the state to share with families the responsibilities of caring for elderly people with major disabilities and to the way in which these responsibilities tend to fall on women.

We have taken a sympathetic view of the policy of 'community care', but point out that practical, financial and emotional support for carers is still inadequate.

We hope this book might contribute in a small way to the increasing interest being shown in the problem of dementia by the general public, as well as being of practical help to those caring for sufferers.

Appendices

Appendix I **Some useful organisations and addresses**

THE ALZHEIMER'S DISEASE SOCIETY
158/160 Balham High Road
London
SW12 9BN
Tel. 081 675 6557/8/9/0
The Alzheimer's Disease Society is a relatively new and energetic organisation dedicated to increasing public awareness of dementia, encouraging research into causes and supporting carers. Local branches exist in most parts of the UK.

AGE CONCERN ENGLAND
60 Pitcairn Road
Mitcham
Surrey
CR4 3LL
Tel. 081 640 5431
Campaigns on behalf of elderly people and also provides many services such as day care, sitting services and transport. Such services may be available in your area.

DISABLED LIVING FOUNDATIONS
380-384 Harrow Road
London
W9 1HU
Able to give advice on various aids and supports for disabled people including those with dementia.

HEALTH EDUCATION COUNCIL
78 New Oxford Street
London
WC1A 1AH
Useful booklet and information available often free of charge.

ASSOCIATION OF CARERS
Medway Homes
Balfour Road
Rochester
Kent

ME4 6QU
Tel. 0634 813981

NATIONAL COUNCIL FOR CARERS AND THEIR ELDERLY DEPENDENTS
29 Chilworth Mews
London
W2 3RG
Tel. 071 262 1451
Both these organisations offer support, information and advice. Local self-help groups are available for those caring for a disabled relative.

NATIONAL ASSOCIATION OF CITIZENS' ADVICE BUREAUX
115-123 Pentamille Road
London
N1 9LZ
Tel. 071 621 1624
Will be able to put you in touch with local Citizens' Advice offices where help is available especially on legal and financial matters.

MIND (NATIONAL ASSOCIATION FOR MENTAL HEALTH)
22 Harley Street
London
WIN 2ED
A national pressure group campaigning in the interests of all people with mental disorder. This includes those suffering from dementia.

Appendix II **Progressive relaxation training**

Introduction

The basic idea of relaxation training has been explained in Chapter 8. Before going on the exercises themselves, we will go over a few points concerning how and when to practise relaxation, and then describe the importance of correct breathing.

1 Make relaxation exercises part of your normal daily routine. As we have seen, relaxation is a skill and so needs regular daily practice. Vary the times you do it initially until you find a time (or times) which suit you.

2 Don't worry if the relaxation exercises do not work for you initially. Keep persevering and you will soon be able to do it.

3 Make sure the room you use to do relaxation in is warm, comfortable and quiet. Make sure you are not disturbed; tell the family not to bother you, take the phone off the hook and so on.

4 The exercises involve tensing the various muscles, so take care when you are tensing them not to overdo it and strain the muscles. Concentrate most of your effort on the relaxation.

5 You can use relaxation in your day-to-day life by learning to recognise how tense you are in various situations, at work and at home, and then relaxing yourself. Even if you are just sitting watching TV, be aware of tension creeping into various muscles, shoulder, neck and stomach muscles especially, and then relax those muscles.

6 People who experience higher than necessary tension levels tend also to be overactive, doing things more hurriedly and rushing about throughout the day. Learn to change this habit by slowing yourself down and taking things more easily (not easy if this has become a real habit, but remember all habits can be broken!).

7 Try to arrange to do the relaxation exercises after having done some physical exercise, as your muscles are then naturally prepared for relaxation.

8 Massage can be a very useful approach in dealing with tension, so it will probably be worthwhile arranging to have massage sessions from a qualified practitioner and/or by learning techniques from self-instructional books which you and a partner can then practise.

BREATHING EXERCISES

The technique of relaxation has two related parts:
1 Breathing exercises
2 Muscular relaxation

The two parts are incorporated in the following exercises but firstly you should bear in mind the importance of correct breathing as you do the exercises. When people become very anxious they invariably breathe rapidly. This rapid breathing serves to intensify various physical signs such as heart rate and dizziness. In fact, people often bring on anxiety attacks by starting to breathe very quickly. People may have told you to 'take deep breaths' to reduce the tension, but in fact this will worsen it if you take too many deep breaths. It is often helpful in anxiety-provoking situations to take one deep breath, then hold if for a few seconds, then slowly let the breath out, relaxing as you do so. Once you have done this aim at breathing slowly and gently. You may find this easier by concentrating on relaxing your stomach muscles as you breathe out. This is because if you are tense the powerful stomach muscles constrict the lower half of your lungs, and this leads to rapid 'shallow' breathing. So, as you breathe out, concentrate on relaxing, the stomach muscles in particular, and when you breathe in again, breathe air firstly into the bottom of the lungs (pushing your stomach outwards) and then into the rest of the lungs.

Finally, remember that correct breathing is a vitally important part of relaxation training, even though it may seem as though it is something which is so natural that it doesn't require attention. When you learn to be aware of the tension-worsening aspects of your breathing pattern, and replace it with a slow, regular, relaxation-inducing breathing pattern, you will have learned one of the keys to relaxation.

PROGRESSIVE MUSCLE RELAXATION TRAINING EXERCISES

Relaxation of arms (time 4-5 min.)

Settle back as comfortably as you can. Let yourself relax to the best of your ability. ... Now, as you relax like that, clench your right fist, just clench your fist tighter and tighter, and study the tension as you do so. Keep it clenched and feel the tension in your right fist, hand, forearm...

And now relax. Let the fingers of your right hand become loose, and observe the contrast in your feelings... Now, let yourself go and try to become more relaxed all over... Once more, clench your right fist really tight ... hold it, and notice the tension again ...

Now let go, relax, let your fingers straighten out, and you notice the difference once more ... Now repeat that with your left fist. Clench your left fist while the rest of your body relaxes, clench the fist tighter and feel the tension ...

And now relax. Again enjoy the contrast ... Repeat that more than once, clench the left fist, tight and tense ...

Now do the opposite of tension, relax and feel the difference. Continue relaxing like that for a while ... Clench both fists tighter and tighter, both fists now tense, forearms tense, study the sensations ...

And relax. Straighten out your fingers and feel that relaxation. Continue relaxing your hands and forearms more and more ... Now bend your elbows and tense your biceps, tense them harder and study the tension feelings ...

Now, straighten out your arms, let them relax and feel the difference again. Let the relaxation develop ... Once more, tense your biceps; hold the tension and observe it carefully ...

Straighten the arms and relax; relax to the best of your ability ... Each time, pay close attention to your feelings when you tense up and when you relax. Now straighten your arms and press your hands together so that you feel most tension in the triceps muscles along the back of your arms. Stretch your arms and press your hands together and feel the tension ...

And now relax. Get your arms back into a comfortable position. Let the relaxation proceed on its own. The arms should feel comfortably heavy as you allow them to relax ... Straighten the arms once more so that you feel the tension in the triceps muscles; straighten them. Feel that tension ...

And relax. Now concentrate on pure relaxation in the arms without any tension. Get your arms comfortable and let them relax further and further. Continue relaxing your arms even further. Even when your arms seem fully relaxed, try to go that extra bit further; try to achieve deeper and deeper levels of relaxation.

Relaxation of facial area with neck, shoulders and upper back (time 4-5 min.)

Let all your muscles go loose and heavy. Just settle back quietly and comfortably. Wrinkle up your forehead now; wrinkle it tighter ...

And now stop wrinkling your forehead, relax and smooth it out. Picture the entire forehead and scalp becoming smoother as the relaxation increases ... Now frown and crease your brows and study the tension ...

Let go of the tension again. Smooth out the forehead once more ... Now close your eyes tighter and tighter ... Feel the tension ...

And relax your eyes. Keep your eyes closed, gently, comfortably, and notice the relaxation... Now clench your jaws, bite your teeth together. Study the tension throughout the jaws ...

Relax your jaws now. Let your lips part slightly ... Appreciate the relaxation ... Now press your tongue hard against the roof of your mouth. Look for tension ...

Now let your tongue return to a comfortable and relaxed position ... Now purse your lips, press your lips together tighter and tighter ...

Relax the lips. Note the contrast between tension and relaxation. Feel the relaxation all over your face, all over your forehead and scalp, eyes, jaws, lips, tongue and throat. The relaxation progresses further and further ...

Now attend to your neck muscles. Press your head back as far as it can go and feel the tension in the neck. Roll it to the right and feel the tension shift; now roll it to the left. Straighten your head and bring it forward, press your chin against your chest.

Let your head return to a comfortable position and study the relaxation. Let the relaxation develop ... Shrug your shoulders, right up. Hold the tension ...

Drop your shoulders and feel the relaxation. Neck and shoulders relaxed ... Shrug your shoulders again and move them around. Bring your shoulders up and forward and back. Feel the tension in your shoulders and in your upper back.

Drop your shoulders once more and relax. Let the relaxation spread deep into the shoulders, right into your back muscles. Relax your neck and throat, and your jaws and other facial areas as the pure relaxation takes over and grows deeper ... deeper ... even deeper.

Relaxation of chest, stomach and lower back (time 4-5 min.)

Relax your entire body to the best of your ability. Feel the comfortable heaviness that accompanies relaxation. Breathe easily and freely in and out. Notice how the relaxation increases as you exhale ... As you breathe out just feel that relaxation ... Now breathe right in and fill your lungs. Inhale deeply and hold your breath. Study the tension ...

Now exhale, let the walls of your chest grow loose and push the air out automatically. Continue relaxing and breathe freely and gently. Feel the relaxation and enjoy it ... With the rest of your body as relaxed as possible, fill your lungs again. Breathe in deeply and hold it again ...

Now, breathe out and appreciate the relief. Just breathe normally. Continue relaxing your chest and let the relaxation spread to your back, shoulders, neck and arms. Just let go ... And enjoy the relaxation. Now pay attention to your abdominal muscles, your stomach area. Tighten your stomach muscles, make your abdomen hard. Notice the tension ...

And relax. Let the muscles loosen and notice the contrast ... Once more, press and tighten your stomach muscles. Hold the tension and study it ...

And relax. Notice the general well-being that comes with relaxing your stomach ... Now draw your stomach in, pull the muscles right in and feel the tension this way ...

Now relax again. Let your stomach out. Continue breathing normally and easily and feel the massaging action all over your chest and stomach. Now pull your stomach in again and hold the tension ... Now push out and tense your muscles like that. Hold the tension ... Once more pull in and feel the tension ...

Now relax your stomach fully. Let the tension dissolve as the relaxation grows deeper. Each time you breathe out, notice the rhythmic relaxation both in your lungs and in your stomach. Notice how your chest and stomach relax more and more ... Try to let go of all contractions anywhere in your body ... Now direct your attention to your lower back. Arch up your back, make your lower back quite hollow, and feel the tension along your spine ...

And settle down comfortably again relaxing the lower back ... Just arch your back up and feel the tensions as you do so. Try to keep the rest of your body as relaxed as possible. Try to localise the tension throughout your lower back area ...

Relax once more, relaxing further and further. Relax your lower back, relax your upper back, spread the relaxation to your stomach, chest, shoulders, arms and facial area. Relax these parts further and further and further and even deeper.

Relaxation of hips, thighs and calves followed by complete body relaxation

Let go of all tensions and relax ... Now flex your buttocks and thighs. Flex your thighs by pressing down your heels as hard as you can ...

Relax and note the difference ... Straighten your knees and flex you thigh muscles again. Hold the tension ...

Relax your hips and thighs. Allow the relaxation to proceed on its own ... Press your feet and toes downwards, away from your face, so that your calf muscles become tense. Study that tension ...

Relax your feet and calves ... This time, bend your feet towards your face so that you feel tension along your shins. Bring your toes right up ...

Relax again ... Keep relaxing for a while ... Now let yourself relax further all over. Relax your feet, ankles, calves and shins, knees, thighs, buttocks and hips. Feel the heaviness of your lower body as you relax still further ... Now spread the relaxation to your stomach, waist, lower back. Let go more and more. Feel that relaxation all over. Let it proceed to your upper back, chest, shoulder and arms and right to the tips of your fingers. Keep relaxing more and more deeply. Make sure that no tension has crept into your throat; relax your neck and your jaws and all your facial muscles. Keep relaxing your whole body like that for a while. Let yourself relax.

Now you can deepen your level of relaxation by concentrating on breathing. Take one deep breath ... Hold it for a few seconds ... And then slowly let it out. Feel all the remaining tension draining away from your muscles as you do so. Carry on breathing slowly and gently. Each time you exhale relax all your muscles, the stomach muscles particularly. When you exhale, you don't need to use any muscles at all, so concentrate on letting go of tension as you breathe out.

Carry on relaxing like this for as long as you wish.

Appendix III **Suggestions for further reading**

The following are examples of official and semi-official reports published by successive governments and government agencies. They provide a background to the emerging policy of 'community care' for elderly people. The latest, and potentially most important, report is the *Caring for People* white paper which has been published at the time of our going to press (November 1989).

1 *Growing Older,* Cmnd 8173. HMSO, London, 1981.
2 *A Happier Old Age,* HMSO, London, 1978.
3 *Elderly People in the Community: Their Service Needs,* HMSO, London, 1983.
  These publications contain the policy statements of successive governments on the community care of the elderly.

4 *Who Cares for the Carers? Opportunities for Those Caring for the Elderly and Handicapped,* Equal Opportunities Commission, Manchester, 1982.
  This official publication draws attention to the needs of those who effectively provide community care, the vast majority of whom are female relatives.

5 *The Rising Tide: Developing Services for Mental Illness in Old Age,* Health Advisory Service, London, 1982.
  Describes the range of psychiatric services which should ideally be in place in each health district in order for the needs of elderly people with dementia to be effectively met.

6 *Caring for People: Community Care in the Next Decade and Beyond,* HMSO, London, 1989.

For greater understanding of the position of elderly people within society we suggest
7 Phillipson, C. and Walker, A. (eds): *Ageing and Social Policy – A Critical Assessment,* Gower Press, Aldershot, 1986.

The reality of residential care for elderly people and especially those with dementia is well described and analysed in the following two books.
8 Booth, T., *Home Truths: Old People's Homes and the Outcome of Care,* Gower Press, Aldershot, 1985.

9 Willcocks, D., Peace, S. and Kelleher, L., *Private Lives in Public Places*, Tavistock, London, 1987.

Readers who would like a more thorough account of how the behavioural approach can be used to help people with dementia are directed to

10 Pinkstad, E. and Linsk, N., *Care of the Elderly: A Family Approach*, Pergamon Press, Oxford, 1984.

Other books specifically giving advice on how to care for a person with dementia are

11 Mace, N. and Robins, P., *The 36-Hour Day: Caring at Home for Elderly People*, Age Concern/Hodder & Stoughton, Sevenoaks, Kent, 1985.
and

12 Murphy, E., *Dementia and Mental Illness in the Old*, Papermac, (Macmillan), London, 1986.

The management of incontinence receives particular attention in

13 Mandelstom, D., *Incontinence and its Management: A Guide to the Understanding of a Very Common Complaint*, Heinemann Health Books for the Disabled Living Foundation, London, 1981.

For those who wish to acquaint themselves with the research into the causes of dementia, a good summary is

14 *Dementia in Later Life: Research and Action*, Report of WHO Scientific Group, Technical Report Series 730, World Health Organisation, Geneva, 1986.

Finally for those unsure of their rights to benefits and of the legal issues relating to the care of a person with dementia, we suggest

15 *Your Rights* for Pensioners by Age Concern, which is an annual publication containing advice for elderly people on state benefits.

16 Norman Alison, *Rights and Risks*, The Centre for Policy on Ageing, London, 1980. Contains information on compulsory care, consent to treatment and other legal issues.

Select glossary

ALZHEIMER'S DISEASE: A disease of the brain first identified by a Dr Alois Alzheimer in 1907. It is the commonest form of dementia at all ages. About 2 out of 3 of all dementia suffers have Alzheimer's disease.

COMPUTERISED AXIAL TOMOGRAPHY: Equipment which helps in the diagnosis of brain disease. It allows the brain to be scanned by X-ray pictures of the head which are analysed by computer to get a picture of what is happening in the brain.

DELIRIUM: Confusion arising suddenly, usually in connection with a physical illness of the body such as a chest or urinary infection. Also known as an acute confusional state.

DEMENTIA: A long-term impairment of memory and thinking which arises gradually because of a disease of the brain such as Alzheimer's disease. (Also known as a chronic confusional state).

DEPRESSION: A disorder of mood which in some severe cases appears very like the effects of dementia. However, depression is treatable and is not a true dementia in that there is no underlying disease of the brain.

CORTEX: The outer layers of the brain where many of our most human capacities and characteristics are located.

ENLARGED PROSTATE GLAND: Gland at the base of the bladder in men which when enlarged causes difficulty in the passing of urine.

HALLUCINATIONS: Seeing things which are not there.

HIPPOCAMPUS: Small horse-shaped structure deep in the brain which has a vital function in co-ordinating memory and which is damaged in Alzheimer's disease.

HUNTINGTON'S CHOREA: A rare and purely inherited disease characterised by sudden jerky movements.

HYPERTENSION: High blood pressure.

HYPOTHERMIA: Decrease in body temperature to dangerously low levels.

JAKOB CREUTZFELDT DISEASE: A very rare dementia which runs a very rapid course (3-9 months in 50% of cases). Thought to be caused by an infective agent which can incubate in the body over a long period of time ('slow virus').

MULTI-INFARCT DEMENTIA: A dementia caused by multiple small strokes which produces small areas of dead tissue in the brain.

NEUROFIBRILLARY TANGLES: Wool-like tangles in the neurons

found in the brains of Alzheimer's disease sufferers.

NEURON: Nerve cell which is the basic building block of the brain and central nervous system.

NORMAL PRESSURE HYDROCEPHALUS: Abnormal flow of spinal fluid.

NEURO-TRANSMITTER: Chemical substance in the brain which allows nerve cells (neurons) to communicate with each other. There are many different neurotransmitters in the brain.

PICK'S DISEASE: A rare form of dementia first noted by Dr A. Pick in 1892. It differs from Alzheimer's disease in that in the early stages changes in personality rather than memory are often evident.

PELVIC FLOOR INSUFFICIENCY: Inadequate control in women of muscles enabling them to control passing of urine.

SENILE DEMENTIA: The term used for dementia in older people (65 years plus). Most of the brains of these older people show signs of Alzheimer's disease. For this reason the term Alzheimer's disease is used to cover dementia in people of all ages.

SENILE PLAQUES: Small island-like areas of diseased neurons found in the brains of sufferers from Alzheimer's disease. This is a type of scarring of the brain caused by the illness.

TRANQUILLISER: Drug used to reduce overall activity, restlessness and agitation. Not a specific cure for any specific problem.

TRANSIENT ISCHAEMIC ATTACK: Short-lived disability lasting only a few minutes or hours, caused by a temporary disruption in blood supply to the brain.